Passing Calculations Tests for Nursing Students

Second Edition

Susan Starkings and Larry Krause

Los Angeles | London | New Delhi
Singapore | Washington DC

Learning Matters
An imprint of SAGE Publications Ltd
1 Oliver's Yard
55 City Road
London EC1Y 1SP

SAGE Publications Inc.
2455 Teller Road
Thousand Oaks, California 91320

SAGE Publications India Pvt Ltd
B 1/I 1 Mohan Cooperative Industrial Area
Mathura Road
New Delhi 110 044

SAGE Publications Asia-Pacific Pte Ltd
3 Church Street
#10-04 Samsung Hub
Singapore 049483

Editor: Alex Clabburn
Development editor: Caroline Sheldrick
Production controller: Chris Marke
Project management: Diana Chambers
Marketing manager: Tamara Navaratnam
Cover design: Wendy Scott
Typeset by: Kelly Winter
Printed by: MPG Printgroup, UK

First published 2010
Second edition published 2013

Library of Congress Control Number: 2013930269

British Library Cataloguing in Publication data

A catalogue record for this book is available from
the British Library

ISBN 978 1 44625 641 1
ISBN 978 1 44625 642 8 (pbk)

MIX
Paper from
responsible sources
FSC
www.fsc.org   FSC® C018575

Contents

Foreword

Nurses are expected to have many different skills; in one minute they are practising the art of emotionally supporting and caring for a patient in distress and in the next they turn to science and mathematical skills to calculate medications. Numeracy is one of those essential ingredients in a nurse's repertoire of skills and this text concentrates on honing the skills nurses need in the basic medicines calculations that are required to assist in the care and treatment of their patients.

You will find in this updated text extremely clear and easy-to-follow instructions to revise, or learn from scratch, the methods you will need to calculate medications, work out metric conversions, fluid balance and intravenous infusions. There is a self-test to guide your learning and a final chapter that helps you prepare for tests and examinations. The text itself is a tonic to take away the panic of drug calculations!

The authors, Susan Starkings and Larry Krause, will provide you with scenarios and case studies to help give context to the situations you will encounter in drugs calculations. It will not give you, however, the detailed pharmacological knowledge or rationales for treating with medications or calculating volumes and quantities. This knowledge is also a fundamental ingredient of managing the care of patients. For this you will need to read further texts in the series on medicines managements; this will provide you with that essential underpinning knowledge to enable you to integrate mathematics with your therapeutic role in care.

I know you will gain confidence and competence from reading and working through the superbly well-written exercises in this text. Good luck with your examinations and your improved numeracy skills, which will add another feature to your growing portfolio of practice skills.

Shirley Bach
Series Editor

Acknowledgements

The publisher and authors would like to thank Heather Short, RGN, Dip/DN, BSc (Hons), MEd, Senior Lecturer, University of the West of England, Bristol, and Mr Patrick Saintas, Principal Lecturer, Faculty of Health and Social Sciences, School of Nursing and Midwifery, University of Brighton, for their helpful comments on early drafts of the first edition of this book.

Guide to the companion website accompanying this book

The companion website that accompanies this book provides students with ready-to-use learning resources. They are free of charge and are designed to maximise the learning experience.

 www.sagepub.co.uk/starkings2e

Extra questions and activities

When it comes to calculations, it is impossible to ever have too much practice. The authors have provided a range of extra questions so that you can get additional preparation on any topics you are not yet confident about.

Interactive glossary

The book introduces a number of important common terms and to help you learn and memorise these an interactive glossary has been produced that you can work through to check your understanding.

Pull-out section from the back of the book

At the back of the book there is a page with some handy formulas for your reference. We have made this available as a pdf which you can download to whatever device you like so that you can access this extremely useful tool at all times.

Useful weblinks

There is a huge amount of helpful information available on the internet that will help you to improve your mathematics and numeracy skills and the authors have provided a range of recommendations for you.

Introduction

The aim of this book is to put the calculations required for nursing into the practical contexts that you should encounter during your training. It was written after seeing, over many years, the problems that student nurses commonly encounter. The text aims to address these problems using realistic examples.

Book structure

The book has been designed to supplement your nursing studies and to be used for self-study. The first chapter contains a diagnostic test. We suggest that you try out this test first to identify which areas of numeracy you need help with. Then work through the chapters relevant to the area(s) identified: when you feel that you have understood these areas, re-do the diagnostic test and compare the results from your first attempt. Chapter 2 contains the basic arithmetic required for nursing calculations. Chapter 3 shows you how to convert from one metric quantity to another, and Fluid Balance Charts are covered in Chapter 4. A simple and effective method to calculate the correct drug dosage in liquid, tablet or capsule form is in Chapter 5. How to calculate the required rate of an intravenous drip rate using the most commonly found equipment values is covered in Chapter 6, while calculating children's drug doses is covered in Chapter 7.

Finally, Chapter 8 will help you prepare for any calculations tests you might be taking, and includes advice on how to prepare for the test, revision questions and tips on common errors to avoid.

Learning features

Each chapter begins with an outline of what is covered in the chapter. There is also information on how the chapter content will help you meet the requirements of the Nursing and Midwifery Council (NMC) *Standards for Pre-registration Nursing Education* (NMC, 2010) and Essential Skills Clusters (ESCs). These are a set of requirements about what skills and competencies you will need to demonstrate in order to become a registered nurse; your nursing programme will have been designed around them. There are specific requirements for medicines calculations and numeracy: these are highlighted in each chapter so that you can see how you are progressing towards achieving these requirements.

Case studies and scenarios are introduced throughout the text to illustrate the relevant nursing calculations and each chapter has activities, with solutions, for you to try. Useful websites can be found at the end of each chapter. Please note that responsibility for the content of any of the web pages referenced in this text is controlled by third parties.

There is a glossary of terms at the end of the book that provides an interpretation of some of the terminology in the context of the subject of the book. Glossary terms are in **bold** in the first instance they appear.

This book does not cover all nursing calculations, and questions, scenarios and case studies are as realistic as possible but are not related to any real person. To obtain maximum benefit from this book it is suggested that you work through the diagnostic test in Chapter 1 first.

A note on terminology

Please note that it is recommended that micrograms and nanograms should not be abbreviated in practice – that is, using the symbols 'mcg' and 'ng' (*British National Formulary* (BNF) (2010) *BNF* 59. London: BMJ Group/Pharmaceutical Press, available online at www.bnf.org/bnf.) Abbreviated forms of measurements have been used occasionally in this book to save space. Great care should be taken not to confuse mg (milligrams) with mcg (micrograms) and ng (nanograms) as this can lead to errors. However, there may be occasions when you see these abbreviations in books, journal articles or even on patients' prescriptions. You must always follow your Trust/Employer and University policies regarding the approved abbreviations that you are allowed to use.

Chapter 1
Diagnostic assessment

NMC Standards for Pre-registration Nursing Education

At the end of this chapter you should have identified the essential numerical calculations required for the Essential Skills Clusters at the first progression point and entry to the register.

33(1)   Is competent in basic medicine calculations.
33(2)   Is competent in the process of medication-related calculation in nursing field

NMC Essential Skills Clusters

The indicative content outlined in the Essential Skills Cluster on Medicines Management are as follows:

*   Numeracy skills.
*   Drug calculations required to administer medicines safely via appropriate routes including specific requirements for children and other groups.

Chapter aims

By the end of this chapter you will have:

*   completed the diagnostic test;
*   identified areas of numeracy that you need help with from your diagnostic test results;
*   selected the relevant chapter(s) that would be useful to aid your studies.

Introduction

Nurses need to achieve competence in numeracy skills in order to cope safely with calculations. These skills are essential to the safe administration of medications and general nursing calculations involved with patient care for both adults and children. Nurses do not need higher degree qualifications in mathematics, so do not worry. Essential nursing calculations will be covered in this text to help you achieve the skills required for safe nursing practice.

Calculator usage

Most nursing calculations carried out for assessment purposes are usually performed without the use of a calculator so it is important that you can do the calculations manually (on paper) or in your head. It is therefore recommended that the questions in the chapters are answered without the use of a calculator. You can, should you wish, use a calculator to check your answers for the purpose of studying, but carry out the calculations manually first.

Diagnostic test

The purpose of this exercise is to highlight the numeracy and mathematics required for the modern nurse. Attempt the diagnostic test, without using a calculator, to assess your current understanding and mathematical ability. Solutions are provided at the end of this chapter, along with advice on which chapters within this book to refer to for further assistance or revision. Appropriate online resources that you could use to aid your learning further, and for practice purposes, are recommended. The two main websites that have been recommended here are BBC Bitesize and the Higher Education Academy Centre for Excellence in Teaching and Learning Mathcentre website. You may also like to use the Open University OpenLearn website, which gives free access to learning materials.

For this test you do not need any prior knowledge of healthcare or nursing terminology. The aim of the test is for you to ascertain your own numerical and mathematical ability in addition, subtraction, multiplication, division, fractions, decimals, percentages, ratios, factors and metric conversions, all of which will be used throughout your future career as a registered nurse.

This diagnostic test is designed to allow you to determine your current level of mathematical ability; it is not a speed test. Hence you may take as long as you feel necessary to undertake this exercise. It is suggested that you complete the test by yourself to ascertain your own strengths and weaknesses in your numerical and mathematical ability. Seeking assistance at this point will not give you a true indication of your strengths and the areas in need of further revision.

Each section, consisting of ten questions, introduces you, the future registered nurse, to some of the calculations needed to accurately determine the correct amount of medication to be given to your future patients. In later chapters you will use the skills tested here to carry out the more specialised nursing calculations you will use throughout your career.

The questions below cover the maths you need to accurately complete the range of nursing calculations covered in this book as well as those you will see as a registered nurse. At the end of the test, check your answers and make an assessment of where you need to start. Alternatively, you can work through the whole book and come back to the diagnostic test at a later stage.

There is no need for you to worry if you cannot do some of the questions at this stage, since you can work through the book at your own pace to improve your numerical and mathematical ability.

It is your decision what chapter or chapters you wish to work through once you have identified gaps in your skills from your results in the diagnostic test. If you wish to know your percentage score for the test, just add up the number of questions you answered correctly; this number is also the percentage score that you have obtained (because there are 100 questions).

Now work through each section and identify what chapter you need to start with. Work at your own pace, and remember that it is not a speed test.

Addition and subtraction

Calculate the following:

1. $125 + 790 =$
2. $305 + 186 =$
3. $1240 - 750 =$
4. $1065 - 1197 =$
5. $207 + 27 + 127 =$
6. $(416 - 28 + 235) - (278 + 254) =$
7. $(56 - 23) - (34 - 21) =$
8. $276 - 123 - 45 =$
9. $276 - (123 - 45) =$
10. $(789 - 57) - (650 - 245) =$

Addition and subtraction are among the basic numeracy skills essential for nursing calculations, so it is important for you to be able to do these accurately. Should you have any difficulty with addition and subtraction, it is suggested that you start at Chapter 2 (Essential numeracy requirements for nursing) and work your way through this book. You may also like to use the online BBC Bitesize practice material. This website has examples and practice questions for you to try out and check against the solutions. For addition and subtraction, use web pages 1 and 2 listed at the end of this chapter.

These numerical calculations are required for many areas of nursing, especially **Fluid Balance Charts**; see Chapter 4 for examples, scenarios and case studies.

Multiplication and division

Calculate the following:

11.	2.65×1000	16.	0.675×1000
12.	560×2.25	17.	0.032×1000
13.	$575 \div 100$	18.	2.072×100
14.	$12.25 \div 1.75$	19.	$159.7 \div 10$
15.	$2072 \div 8$	20.	$68.86 \div 100$

Should you have any difficulty with multiplication and division, it is suggested that you start at Chapter 2 and work your way through this book. You may also like to use web pages 5 and 6 listed at the end of this chapter.

Multiplication and division are used extensively for the quantity conversions covered in Chapter 3, and in the drug calculations that you will see in Chapter 5. For example, you will need to be able to convert milligrams to micrograms and centimetres to millimetres as part of your routine tasks.

Fractions

Write the following in their simplest form:

21. $\dfrac{25}{75}$ 26. $\dfrac{221}{1768}$

22. $\dfrac{15}{75}$ 27. $\dfrac{375}{1000}$

23. $\dfrac{30}{405}$ 28. $\dfrac{64}{72}$

24. $\dfrac{36}{128}$ 29. $\dfrac{124}{868}$

25. $\dfrac{625}{875}$ 30. $\dfrac{7}{56}$

For drug calculations, the simplification of fractions is an essential skill. Should you have any difficulty with questions 21–30, it is suggested that you start at Chapter 2. For online practice, use web pages 3 (BBC Bitesize) and 16 (Mathcentre) listed at the end of this chapter.

Multiplying and dividing fractions

Solve each of the following, leaving your answer as a fraction in its lowest terms:

31. $\dfrac{14}{100} \times \dfrac{5}{1}$ 34. $\dfrac{3}{12} \div \dfrac{6}{12}$

32. $\dfrac{9}{18} \times \dfrac{18}{81}$ 35. $\dfrac{7}{42} \div \dfrac{14}{21}$

33. $\dfrac{3}{14} \times \dfrac{14}{21}$ 36. $\dfrac{9}{5} \div \dfrac{81}{20}$

continued . . .

37. $\dfrac{4}{24} \div \dfrac{4}{12}$ 39. $\dfrac{3}{16} \div \dfrac{1}{2}$

38. $\dfrac{12}{11} \div \dfrac{36}{22}$ 40. $\dfrac{2}{3} \times \dfrac{3}{6}$

Most of the drug calculations you will be required to perform use these types of calculations. If you have any problems here, start at Chapter 2. For online practice, use web page 4 (BBC Bitesize); for the rules of arithmetic, see web page 18 (Mathcentre) listed at the end of this chapter.

In Chapter 5 you will find examples of drug calculations requiring these types of numerical skills. Children's nursing also requires these skills, and Chapter 7 has examples of child nursing calculations that all nurses, not just children's nurses, should be familiar with.

Decimals and percentages

Write the following as fractions in their simplest form:

41. 0.75   46. $37\frac{1}{2}$ %

42. 0.125   47. 0.0010

43. 10%   48. 0.015

44. 0.35   49. 15%

45. 12.5%   50. 0.02

A drug concentration can be given in the form of a percentage of the total volume available; hence you need to be able to interpret percentages and convert them to fractions in order to calculate the dosage required for your patient. Throughout Chapter 5 (Drug calculations) you will meet examples using this type of numeracy. For example, if you have to dilute a solution, say to clean a wound, then you will need to understand percentages. Fractions and decimals will be covered in Chapter 2; if you find these practice questions difficult, start at this chapter. For online practice you could use web pages 8 and 10 (BBC Bitesize) or 15 and 17 (Mathcentre) listed at the end of this chapter.

Fractions and percentages

Convert each of the following to a decimal:

51. $\dfrac{2}{4}$ 53. $\dfrac{1}{25}$

52. 15%   54. 18%

continued...

55.	$\dfrac{3}{100}$	58.	$\dfrac{7}{1000}$
56.	0.1%	59.	27%
57.	58%	60.	44%

It is essential that you can convert between fractions, percentages and decimals easily and quickly. Decimals will be covered in Chapter 2; if you find these questions difficult, it is advised that you start at this chapter. Downloadable booklets on fractions, decimals and percentages can be found on web pages 15, 16 and 17 (Mathcentre); web page 10 (BBC Bitesize) is also a good online resource with which to supplement your study.

Units of measurement

Find the equivalent metric measure for each of the following:

The use of the unit of measure is a critical part of the answer.

61. 0.35g = ? mg
62. 0.5mg = ? micrograms
63. 290ml = ? litres
64. 875g = ? kg
65. 0.01 microgram = ? nanograms
66. ? g = 1750mg
67. ? kg = 4250g
68. ? litres = 2050ml
69. ? mg = 5.05g
70. 3.75 mole = ? millimoles

Please see note on page 2 concerning the use of abbreviations.

Questions 61–70 test your knowledge of the units generally used in clinical medicine and by nurses in the giving of medications. It is vital that you can accurately convert from one unit to another; this is required for many of the drug calculations that you will carry out as part of your duties as a registered nurse.

Conversion from one unit to another is one of the most common sources of error in nursing. This can be dangerous: an overdose could lead to further health complications or prove fatal, while an under dose may impede a patient's recovery as the medication may not function correctly. Chapter 3 (Quantity conversions for nurses) covers the conversions most commonly used in nursing calculations; if you made any errors in the above questions, Chapter 3 would make an ideal starting point. For online practice, see web page 14 (BBC Bitesize).

Other calculations involving conversions include the calculation of intravenous drip rates; in Chapter 6, for example, a conversion from hours to minutes is used. For online practice with units of time, see web page 7 (BBC Bitesize) listed at the end of this chapter. However, before attempting Chapter 6, make sure you have covered and understood the processes and procedures covered in Chapter 3.

Ratios and factors

Convert the following ratios to percentages:

71. 1 in 4
72. 1:4
73. 1 in 100
74. 1 in 25
75. 1:49

Work out the following factors:

76. Which of the numbers 2, 3, 4, 8 are factors of 124?
77. What are the prime factors of 42?
78. The prime factors of 35 are ... ?
79. What are the common prime factors of 15 and 75?
80. What are the common prime factors of 24 and 42?

You need to understand the ways in which the strength or dilution of a solution is written on the labels of any medication that you deal with in practice. Liquid solutions may be labelled with a ratio (or proportion of volume): for example, '1:1000 adrenaline' is a typical format that you might see on the hospital ward. Chapter 2 explains the use of ratios; for online practice, see web page 11 (BBC Bitesize); for practical examples of ratios, see Chapter 5 (Drug calculations) and Chapter 6 (Calculating intravenous rates).

It is beneficial to know what the factors of numbers are because this makes cancelling down, which is used in drug dosage calculations, easier. Familiarisation with factors will improve your speed at all types of nursing calculations, especially when working without a calculator, as is required for your formal assessments. Most of the formal assessments you have to do as part of your training will be timed and hence a certain amount of speed is required. For online practice in number factors, see web page 12 (BBC Bitesize).

Rounding decimals

Round the following to one decimal place:

81. 10.3756
82. 1.24
83. 200.2781
84. 1000.8491
85. 123.41
86. 456.06
87. 2.7358
88. 0.9733
89. 0.374
90. 0.614

Some of the nursing calculations you do will not give a whole number answer, and you will need to round the answer to an appropriate degree of accuracy: to a whole number or to a certain number of decimal places. Rounding of numbers will be covered in Chapter 2; online practice can be found on web pages 13 (BBC Bitesize) and 19 and 20 (OpenLearn).

The final ten questions in this diagnostic test are 'word questions'; they are closer in style and type to the nursing calculations you will have to do during your training. In case study tests, a scenario will be given in a written format and it is the student's or trainee's task to understand and obtain all the relevant information required to calculate the answer; case studies are presented throughout this book so that you can practise these skills. Some trainee nurses find this style easier as the questions are more realistic; however, the numeracy required to undertake them is similar to the previous questions in this test.

Word questions

The use of the unit of measure is a critical part of the answer.

91. Write the following number in figures: seven thousand, two hundred and fifty-one.
92. How much is 5% of 400g?
93. What is two litres in millilitres?
94. In a ward of 25 patients, five of them are under one year of age. What percentage of these patients is over one year old?
95. Complete: 1.5 gram = ? milligram
96. How many minutes are there in three and a half hours?
97. Mrs Hall is ordered 48mg of phenobarbitone to be taken orally. Tablets in your medicine cabinet are 16mg tablets. How many tablets does Mrs Hall need?
98. Mr Hart should have a **fluid intake** of two litres. He has drunk the following: 275ml of tea twice, 300ml of coffee, 200 ml of orange juice and 180ml of water. How much more fluid should Mr Hart take to reach the two litres required?
99. Miss Reeta Patel must have nil by mouth for 10 hours before her operation, which is scheduled for 8:30 a.m. At what time must you start her nil by mouth? (Answer in 24-hour time format.)
100. Mr Bumbler was given 150ml per hour for $6\frac{1}{3}$ hours. How many ml in total did he receive?

If you find these ten questions difficult, re-read them and pick out the relevant information required for the calculations. For online help with units of time, see web page 7 (BBC Bitesize) listed at the end of this chapter.

Hint … There are lots of context-based questions throughout this book to give you the practice you need. Read on and spend some time on the areas that you have identified as problematic. Read the chapters you have identified as most relevant and work through the scenarios, case studies and practice questions included.

If you have had few problems with the above questions, you might prefer to start at Chapter 4 and work your way through the following chapters in order to make sure you

continued . . .

can do the nursing calculations covered accurately. You can always refer back to an earlier chapter should you need to refresh your memory on any aspect of numeracy. Chapter 2 covers the basic numeracy required to start your nursing calculations.

Answers to the diagnostics test

1. 915
2. 491
3. 490
4. −132

5. 361
6. 91
7. 20

8. 108
9. 198
10. 327

11. 2650
12. 1260
13. 5.75
14. 6.6

15. 259
16. 675
17. 32

18. 207.2
19. 15.97
20. 0.6886

21. $\dfrac{1}{3}$

22. $\dfrac{1}{5}$

23. $\dfrac{2}{27}$

24. $\dfrac{9}{32}$

25. $\dfrac{5}{7}$

26. $\dfrac{1}{8}$

27. $\dfrac{3}{8}$

28. $\dfrac{8}{9}$

29. $\dfrac{1}{7}$

30. $\dfrac{1}{8}$

31. $\dfrac{7}{10}$

32. $\dfrac{1}{9}$

33. $\dfrac{1}{7}$

34. $\dfrac{1}{2}$

35. $\dfrac{1}{4}$

36. $\dfrac{4}{9}$

37. $\dfrac{1}{2}$

38. $\dfrac{2}{3}$

39. $\dfrac{3}{8}$

40. $\dfrac{1}{3}$

41. $\dfrac{3}{4}$

42. $\dfrac{1}{8}$

43. $\dfrac{1}{10}$

44. $\dfrac{7}{20}$

45. $\dfrac{1}{8}$

46. $\dfrac{3}{8}$

47. $\dfrac{1}{1000}$

48. $\dfrac{3}{200}$

49. $\dfrac{3}{20}$

50. $\dfrac{1}{50}$

51. 0.5
52. 0.15
53. 0.04
54. 0.18

55. 0.03
56. 0.001
57. 0.58

58. 0.007
59. 0.27
60. 0.44

61. 350mg
62. 500mcg
63. 0.29L
64. 0.875Kg

65. 10ng
66. 1.75g
67. 4.25Kg

68. 2.05L
69. 5050mg
70. 3750millimole

71. 25%
72. 20%
73. 1%
74. 4%

75. 50%
76. 2, 4
77. 2, 3, 7

78. 5, 7
79. 3 and 5 only
80. 2 and 3 only

81. 10.4
82. 1.2
83. 200.3
84. 1000.8

85. 123.4
86. 456.1
87. 2.7

88. 1.0
89. 0.4
90. 0.6

91. 7251
92. 20g
93. 2000ml
94. 80%

95. 1500mg
96. 210 minutes
97. 3 tablets

98. 770ml
99. 2230hrs
100. 950ml

Useful websites

BBC Bitesize

The BBC Bitesize online resources offer revision material that you can use to enhance your numeracy and mathematical skills. The web pages below have been referenced in this chapter and are accessible free of charge.

1. Addition
   www.bbc.co.uk/schools/ks2bitesize/maths/number/addition/read1.shtml

2. Subtraction
   www.bbc.co.uk/schools/ks2bitesize/maths/number/subtraction/read1.shtml

3. Cancelling fractions
   www.bbc.co.uk/schools/gcsebitesize/maths/number/fractionsrev3.shtml

4. Multiplying and dividing fractions
   www.bbc.co.uk/schools/gcsebitesize/maths/number/fractionsrev22.shtml

5. Long multiplication
   www.bbc.co.uk/schools/gcsebitesize/maths/number/multiplicationdivisionrev1. shtml

6. Long division
   www.bbc.co.uk/schools/gcsebitesize/maths/number/multiplicationdivisionrev2. shtml

7. Units of time
   www.bbc.co.uk/schools/ks2bitesize/maths/shape_space/measures/read7.shtml

8. Decimals
   www.bbc.co.uk/schools/gcsebitesize/maths/number/decimalsrev1.shtml

9. Percentages
   www.bbc.co.uk/schools/gcsebitesize/maths/number/percentagesrev1.shtml

10. Converting fractions and decimals
    www.bbc.co.uk/schools/gcsebitesize/maths/number/fracsdecpersrev1.shtml

11. Ratios
    www.bbc.co.uk/schools/gcsebitesize/maths/number/ratiosrev2.shtml

12. Prime factors
    www.bbc.co.uk/schools/gcsebitesize/maths/number/primefactorsrev1.shtml

13. Rounding decimals
    www.bbc.co.uk/schools/gcsebitesize/maths/number/roundestimaterev2.shtml

14. Converting measurements
    www.bbc.co.uk/schools/gcsebitesize/maths/shapes/measuresrev1.shtml

Mathcentre

Another useful free online resource is the Higher Education Academy Centre for Excellence in Teaching and Learning Mathcentre which offers students quick reference guides, practice and revision materials, video tutorials, workbooks and online practice exercises on many branches of mathematics. For nurses the following areas contain useful extra practice material and have been referenced in this chapter.

15. Decimals
    www.mathcentre.ac.uk/students.php/health/arithmetic/decimals/resources/386

16. Fractions
    www.mathcentre.ac.uk/students.php/health/arithmetic/fractions/resources/

17. Percentages
    www.mathcentre.ac.uk/students.php/health/arithmetic/percentages/resources/

18. Rules of arithmetic
    www.mathcentre.ac.uk/students.php/health/arithmetic/rules/resources/

OpenLearn

The Open University (OU) OpenLearn website gives free access to learning materials from higher education courses. The following pages are relevant to your nursing studies.

19. Numbers, units and arithmetic
    http://labspace.open.ac.uk/course/view.php?id=3434

20. Rounding and estimation
    http://labspace.open.ac.uk/course/view.php?id=3586

 For further activities and other useful material, visit the companion website at
www.sagepub.co.uk/starkings2e

Chapter 2
Essential numeracy requirements for nursing

NMC Standards for Pre-registration Nursing Education

At the end of this chapter you will have covered some of the numerical calculations required for the Essential Skills Clusters by the first and second progression point and for entry to the register.

29(2)   Accurately monitors and records fluid intake and output.
33(1)   Is competent in basic medicines calculations.
33(2)   Is competent in the process of medication-related calculation in nursing field

Chapter aims

By the end of this chapter you should be able to:

- cancel down fractions;
- multiply decimal numbers by other decimal values;
- divide decimals numbers by other decimal values;
- convert fractions to decimals;
- convert decimals to fractions;
- round decimal and fraction values as appropriate;
- convert time fractions and decimals to minutes;
- carry out addition and subtraction.

Introduction

Patients and service users rely on nurses to accurately calculate and administer their medication. Too little could see the patient not recovering in the manner that would be expected; too much could have potentially harmful or fatal consequences.

The numeracy and calculations required of nurses are not difficult once practised and you will not need to use a calculator. Activities are included throughout this book for you to attempt without using a calculator. This chapter will lead you through the best-practice methods of determining the correct answers for all the calculations you will encounter as a successful nurse.

As a nurse you will carry out many calculations, ranging from dosage of medication for your patients to the hydration levels on their Fluid Balance Charts. The mathematics required is not difficult and with practice is readily mastered. If you are worried about the maths you need as a nurse, then you have the right book; throughout this chapter you will see the easiest way in which to overcome your fears of the mathematics needed to become successful. The skills you will learn in this chapter will be used in the other chapters of this book and will be invaluable throughout your nursing career. They will also enable you to pass your drugs calculation tests.

It may seem a challenge to you at the moment but with practice and determination you will become proficient in all elements of the mathematics used in nursing.

One of the first things required is a basic knowledge of multiplication tables. To some people this can be daunting. However, it need not be so as just four numbers are enough to start with. If you know the times tables for the first four **prime numbers**, you can 'cancel down' most numbers.

2   3   5   7

These numbers are the first four prime numbers, meaning they can be divided only by themselves and one. All other numbers can be built by multiplying combinations of prime numbers. Two of the prime numbers listed above are very powerful as they can be used to cancel down three out of every five numbers, no matter how many digits they have.

Hint ...

If a number ends in   0   or   2   or   4   or   6   or   8

Then it is divisible by 2

If a number ends in   0   or   5

Then it is divisible by 5

Cancelling down fractions

When cancelling down a fraction, the numbers on the top and bottom of the fraction must be cancelled by the same value at the same time. You do not have to use the same value each time you cancel and could use different values at different times. The numbers being divided must divide exactly by whatever value you are cancelling down with.

Hint ... When cancelling down a fraction, the numbers on the top and bottom of the fraction must be cancelled by the same value at the same time.

In Chapter 5 (Drug calculations) we look at liquid, tablet and capsule doses; the calculations involved are much simpler if you have cancelled down. For this worked example only part of a drug calculation will be shown.

Worked example

As part of a drug calculation you need to cancel down the following fraction.

$$\frac{375}{675}$$

The fraction ends in 5 on the top and 5 on the bottom, so both numbers are divisible by 5.

$$\frac{375}{675} \div \frac{5}{5} = \frac{75}{135}$$

Again, the numbers on the top and bottom of the fraction can be divided by 5 as they both end in 5.

$$\frac{75}{135} \div \frac{5}{5} = \frac{15}{27}$$

Having cancelled down this far, it is still possible to divide top and bottom. This time you can divide by 3 - this is the only number that both 15 and 27 can be divided by exactly.

$$\frac{15}{27} \div \frac{3}{3} = \frac{5}{9}$$

continued . . . •••

This fraction, five-ninths, is the same as the original fraction and cannot be cancelled any further. It is much easier to use in nursing calculations than the original fraction.

In all the chapters of this book your ability to cancel down will be reviewed time and again; it is a core skill that you will require throughout your career.

In the above worked example, you may have noticed that you could have cancelled down using the factor 25. Provided you are comfortable working with a larger number like this, there is no reason not to do so. Given time, you may even build your confidence and ability levels sufficiently to use numbers like 125. For now, just be aware that $125 = 25 \times 5$, or $125 = 5 \times 5 \times 5$ and so dividing by 125 is the same as dividing by 5 three times in succession. Similarly, in Chapter 5 (Drug calculations) you will see that cancelling down by 16 is the same as dividing by 2 four times in succession, because $2 \times 2 \times 2 \times 2 = 16$. The importance of practice cannot be emphasised enough; the more you do, the better, faster and more accurate you will become at the numeracy skills required as a nurse.

Activity 2.1

Cancel down the following fractions to their simplest form, dividing top and bottom until no further number is exactly divisible into both parts of the fraction.

1. $\dfrac{375}{550}$	2. $\dfrac{625}{890}$	3. $\dfrac{325}{375}$	4. $\dfrac{64}{96}$	5. $\dfrac{42}{96}$	6. $\dfrac{24}{69}$
7. $\dfrac{575}{1275}$	8. $\dfrac{25}{520}$	9. $\dfrac{45}{475}$	10. $\dfrac{54}{181}$	11. $\dfrac{21}{24}$	12. $\dfrac{35}{230}$

Answers to all the activities can be found at the end of the chapter.

Multiplying decimals

Some students become anxious when confronted with numbers containing a decimal point. Nurses need to be able to multiply and divide numbers with a decimal point in either one or both numbers. Just as with the cancelling of fractions, what you need is practice.

> ## Case study
>
> *Catherine works in a mental health clinic where a service user, Maximillian Moreno, has been prescribed 0.375 grams of venlafaxine daily. To ensure there is sufficient stock on hand she has been asked to calculate in grams the amount of venlafaxine required for Maximillian for a 7-day period.*

Catherine has two main options: she can avoid multiplication of a number with a decimal point by converting the amount (0.375 grams) to milligrams (see Chapter 3, Quantity conversions for nurses) and then convert the answer back to grams; or she can multiply 0.375 by 7 and go straight to the answer required.

$$
\begin{array}{r}
0.375 \;\boxed{3} \\
\times\,7 \;\boxed{0} \\
\hline
2625
\end{array}
\qquad
\begin{array}{r}
0.375 \\
\times\,7 \\
\hline
2.625 \\
\end{array}
\qquad
\begin{array}{r}
0.375 \\
\times\,7 \\
\hline
2.625
\end{array}
$$

The placement of the decimal point is often a stumbling block when a multiplication involves decimal points. The easiest way to determine the position of the decimal point in the answer is to count the number of decimal places in the two numbers being multiplied. In the example above you can see that the top number has three decimal places and the bottom number has zero decimal places. By adding these two values together (and in this case getting three) you can find the correct number of decimal places for the answer. Starting to the right of the last digit, count back the correct number of places (in this case, three) and insert the decimal point. In this example the correct answer is 2.625 grams.

Activity 2.2

As part of a stocktake of drugs at Bluebell Care and Respite Centre, you are to calculate the weekly (7-day) requirement in grams of the prescribed drug dosages for the following patients.

1. Sebastian Contina needs to have 0.015g per day
2. Jess Crome needs to have 0.15g per day
3. Steven Gusty needs to have 0.0106g per day

Later on your placement you carry out a similar stocktake at Daffodil Rehabilitation Clinic. Again you need to calculate the weekly (7-day) requirement in grams of drugs for the following patients.

4. Helen Reckit needs to have 0.45g per day
5. Mark Strode needs to have 0.121g per day
6. Alison Barbara needs to have 0.05g per day
7. Falua McTaggart needs to have 0.25g per day
8. Arthur Dat needs to have 5.5g per day
9. Iain Burns needs to have 0.075g per day

Division of decimals

Division by whole numbers

The division of a number containing a decimal point can also be done simply because the decimal point in the number being divided will be placed directly above this number. The solution to the task in the following scenario will show you how it is done.

Scenario

Harold Johnson has been prescribed clemastine fumarate syrup for treatment of his allergic rhinitis. The syrup comes in a bottle containing 75 millilitres. The amount of clemastine fumarate in a bottle of this size is 10.05 milligrams. This is expressed as 10.05mg/75ml on the bottle's label.

You are asked to calculate how many milligrams of clemastine fumarate there are in each millilitre of the syrup. This figure will then be used in later calculations in order to fulfil Mr Johnson's medication requirement.

Given that the bottle contains 75 millilitres, dividing by 75 will reduce the amount to 1 millilitre: any number divided by itself is always 1. The amount of clemastine fumarate in 75 millilitres is 10.05 milligrams. To find the amount of clemastine fumarate in 1ml, you therefore need to divide the drug weight by 75 as well. Making sure that you always divide both the liquid measure and the drug weight by the same number will keep the calculation in balance.

$$75ml \div 75 \qquad 10.05mg \div 75$$

This method of calculating the strength per millilitre will be used throughout your nursing career.

In the above scenario you used 75 to reduce the number of millilitres to 1. In the activity that follows you will practise using different liquid volumes. Divide the liquid measure by the total volume to reduce the amount to 1ml, and divide the drug weight by the same number.

Hint ... Always remember to divide both the liquid measure and the drug amount by the same number to keep the calculation balanced.

There will be times when you are dividing numbers and find that you are not able to divide exactly into every digit of the number, or that a digit is too small to be divided. When this occurs, carry that digit or any remainder over to the next available digit in the number being divided. Should you not be able to divide into a digit, remember to place a zero in the answer to indicate this. This method is shown in the first of the diagrams below. The second shows how you would go on to complete the division. The digits and remainders being carried through are shown using smaller digits, written before the next digit in the number being divided. Always continue until the remainder is zero to obtain the correct answer.

0 0. 1

$75 \overline{)\ 1^{1}0.^{10}0\ 5\ 0}$

0. 1 3 4

$75 \overline{)\ 1^{1}0.^{10}0^{25}5\ 5^{30}0^{0}0}$

So 10.05 divided by 75 is equal to 0.134, which tells you each 1 millilitre of syrup contains 0.134 milligrams of weight of the drug. You will use this type of division throughout your career, for example when calculating drug doses or intravenous flow rates.

Activity 2.3

Calculate the amount of drug weight in 1 millilitre of the following syrup mixtures.

1. 9.6mcg/6ml	2. 56.7mg/7ml	3. 97.5mcg/5ml
4. 1.2g/8ml	5. 1.5mg/4ml	6. 7.04mg/8ml
7. 9.2mcg/4ml	8. 55.055g/55ml	9. 0.072mg/3ml

Division by other decimal values

Should you have to divide a number containing a decimal point by another number that also contains a decimal point, then you need to carry out a preliminary step. Prior to carrying out the division, the number you are dividing by must be made into a whole number. The method of doing this is covered extensively in Chapter 3 (Quantity conversions for nurses) and requires multiplication by 10, 100 or 1000. The number being divided does not need to have its decimal point removed, as seen in the above scenario. However, you must remember to keep things in balance and so you must always multiply both numbers in the calculation by the same value.

Scenario

Mercia James has osteoporosis and will be treated with calcitonin. Mercia's GP has prescribed 0.09 millilitres of calcitonin per day via a nasal spray. The bottle containing the spray contains 3.6 millilitres. Whilst on placement at the surgery you are asked to work out how many doses of calcitonin Mercia will receive from each bottle of nasal spray.

In order to calculate the number of doses, you need to divide the bottle's contents (3.6ml) by the single dose amount (0.09ml). The number you need to divide by has a decimal point and needs to be made into a whole number prior to the division being carried out. Multiplication by 100 will see the dose 0.09 transformed to become 9. (If you need more detail on this method, see Chapter 3.) To maintain the balance in your calculation you need to do the same to the other value and multiply 3.6 by 100, giving a value of 360.

> Hint ... What you do to one side of a calculation you must do to the other.

Now you can divide 360 by 9, obtaining the answer 40. In this case, multiplication by 100 removed the decimal points from both numbers before the division was calculated. However, there is no need to eliminate a decimal point from the number being divided, as shown in the earlier worked example.

Activity 2.4

Work out how many doses of medication can be obtained from the following amounts when divided by the decimal numbers.

1. $8.1 \div 0.9$
2. $1.5 \div 0.05$
3. $0.075 \div 0.0025$
4. $10 \div 2.5$
5. $0.325 \div 0.025$
6. $0.090 \div 0.015$

Converting fractions to decimals

In Chapter 5 (Drug calculations) you will calculate the doses of medications to be given to patients. One of the potential methods of delivery of this dose is by injection. Since syringes are not marked in fractions you will need to convert any drug amount given as a fraction into a decimal number.

Case study

Herminie Derringer has temporal arteritis, a painful condition. Her doctor has prescribed betamethasone to be administered by the intramuscular route. Her nurse, Audrey, has carried out a drug calculation to find the amount of betamethasone injectable suspension to be drawn for the intramuscular injection (IMI). Audrey finds it is $\frac{27}{5}$ millilitres which is $5\frac{2}{5}$ millilitres.

Herminie's treatment requires her medication to be injected and so Audrey needs the answer in decimal format. Hypodermic syringes are always marked in decimal format and never in fractions, so the amount of liquid in every injection given will need to be converted to decimal format for all non-whole number answers. This can be done prior to cancelling ($\frac{27}{5}$ in this scenario) or using the final result ($5\frac{2}{5}$ here). In either case, you obtain the whole number 5; the fraction $\frac{2}{5}$ indicates a remainder of 2 still to be divided by 5.

> Hint ... To convert any fraction to a decimal you divide the top number by the bottom number.

In this example the top number in the fraction ($\frac{2}{5}$ or $\frac{27}{5}$) does not have a decimal point, so you need to place one directly behind the last digit. You can now divide the top number by the bottom number to find the decimal value.

$$
\begin{array}{r}
0\,.\,4 \\
\hline
5\,\big|\,2\,.^{2}0\ ^{0}0
\end{array}
\qquad\qquad
\begin{array}{r}
5\,.\,4 \\
\hline
5\,\big|\,2\,^{2}7\,.^{2}0\ ^{0}0
\end{array}
$$

When the fraction $\frac{2}{5}$ is converted to a decimal the result is 0.4, which is then added to the whole number 5 to give the final answer, 5.4 millilitres.

If you choose to convert to a decimal from the fraction $\frac{27}{5}$ you should obtain the answer 5.4ml in one step. Notice that both answers are the same, and accurate.

So for Herminie's IMI, Audrey will need to draw up 5.4 millilitres of betamethasone.

Activity 2.5

These twelve fractions are drug doses that you have calculated for patients. Now you need to convert the results to decimal answers, as all the medications are to be injected.

1. $\dfrac{13}{.4}$ 2. $\dfrac{10}{8}$ 3. $\dfrac{22}{4}$ 4. $\dfrac{7}{4}$ 5. $\dfrac{15}{4}$ 6. $\dfrac{26}{4}$

7. $\dfrac{17}{8}$ 8. $\dfrac{34}{8}$ 9. $\dfrac{17}{4}$ 10. $\dfrac{12}{5}$ 11. $\dfrac{21}{10}$ 12. $\dfrac{27}{5}$

Converting decimals to fractions

There will be times when an order is given to a nurse as a decimal, but it would be quicker to complete the task using a fraction, as in the following scenario.

Scenario

Athol Burnett has had a fall from his bicycle and grazed his lower arm and elbow. His injury is not thought to be serious but may require sutures. Prior to Athol's assessment by the Charge Nurse, you have been asked to prepare an iodine solution to clean the wound to remove any loose skin. The solution strength required is 0.2 parts iodine mixed with sterile water.

Athol's injury is to be cleaned using a solution you must prepare. The solution strength is to be 0.2 parts iodine mixed with sterile water. Before you can calculate the amounts required you will need to convert 0.2 to a fraction. This fraction will then show what proportion of the total will be iodine in the mixed solution.

The conversion process is among the easiest you will encounter. To write the decimal as a fraction, use the decimal as the numerator (or top digit/s); the denominator (or bottom digit/s) will be a multiple of 10 (10, 100, 1000 . . .) and can be found by counting the number of decimal places.

In the scenario, Athol's mixture was 0.2 and so the numerator will be 2. Notice that the decimal point has now been dropped. Since the decimal has just one place, there will be one zero in the denominator.

As a fraction 0.2 is $\frac{2}{10}$, which can be cancelled down to $\frac{1}{5}$.

This fraction will allow you to mix the solution to clean Athol's wounds. Since the order was for 0.2 iodine solution and you have now calculated this to be $\frac{1}{5}$, you know that any solution used is to be $\frac{1}{5}$ iodine plus $\frac{4}{5}$ sterile water.

> Hint ... To convert from a fraction to a decimal, use the decimal digits as the numerator, and the number 1 followed by as many zeros as decimal places for the denominator.

Activity 2.6

Convert the following decimals to fractions in their simplest or lowest form.

1. 0.50	2. 0.25	3. 0.375	4. 0.08
5. 0.044	6. 0.04	7. 0.125	8. 0.075
9. 0.010	10. 0.072	11. 0.200	12. 0.875

Rounding decimals and fractions

When you are calculating the flow rate of an intravenous infusion for your patient (as in Chapter 6, Calculating intravenous rates), the answer needs to be a whole number because a droplet cannot be successfully divided. You therefore need to be able to round to the nearest whole number.

Scenario

Following a surgical procedure your patient, Nicola Burke, is to have an intravenous infusion (IV). You have accurately calculated the flow rate using the formula from Chapter 6 and found it to be $41\frac{2}{3}$ or, as a decimal, 41.6 drops per minute. You must now determine the correct number of drops per minute.

Without the correct flow rate, Nicola could receive her IV infusion too quickly, or may not receive her total medication in the prescribed time period. Either case could have serious consequences.

To decide whether to round up or down, simply judge if the fraction or decimal has reached or passed half way. If your answer is a decimal, look at the first number after the decimal point. If this number is 5 or greater, then the number before the decimal point should be increased to the next whole number. The decimal point and every number beyond it are then deleted.

If your answer is a whole number plus a fraction, look at the fraction. If the numerator (top number) of the fraction is half or more of the denominator (bottom number), then the whole number should be increased to the next number. The fraction is then deleted from your answer.

For answers where the decimal or fractions do not reach half way or greater, then the decimal or fraction is simply deleted from the answer and the whole number is not changed.

Hint ... If the decimal is 0.5 or larger, or the fraction $\frac{1}{2}$ or larger, then the whole number value increases to the next whole number value and the decimal or fraction is deleted. If the decimal or fraction is less than half, the whole number value remains unchanged and the decimal or fraction is deleted.

In the scenario above, Nicola's IV flow rate was calculated at $41\frac{2}{3}$ or 41.6 drops per minute. The fraction $\frac{2}{3}$ is greater than $\frac{1}{2}$ and the decimal 0.6 is greater than 0.5. So when you set the flow rate for Nicola's IV you will set it at 42 drops/minute.

In preparation for later chapters in this book, attempt the following activity on rounding of fractions and decimals.

Activity 2.7

Round each of the following values to the nearest whole number.

1. 1.7
2. $4\frac{19}{35}$
3. 11.92
4. $2\frac{6}{7}$
5. $59\frac{5}{8}$
6. $49\frac{7}{15}$
7. 39.6
8. $25\frac{3}{5}$
9. 28.49
10. 60.4
11. $21\frac{8}{10}$
12. 63.7
13. $24\frac{14}{29}$
14. 17.18
15. 9.9

Converting time fractions and decimals to minutes

There will be times when the number of hours over which a medication or treatment is to be given is not in whole hours. For example, on your placement you may encounter a patient having chemotherapy whose treatment does not take an exact number of whole hours.

Details of how to calculate the length of time taken are covered in Chapter 6 (Calculating intravenous rates); here we shall concentrate on the conversion of the time fraction.

To convert a time fraction to a number of minutes, multiply the fraction by 60. Since there are 60 minutes in one hour, this will give the exact number of minutes equal to the fraction of an hour. For Rosie this means $\frac{1}{3} \times 60$ which you can cancel down using skills learnt earlier in this chapter.

$$\frac{1}{\cancel{3}} \times \frac{\cancel{60}}{1} = \frac{1}{1} \times \frac{20}{1} = \frac{20}{1} = 20 \text{ minutes}$$

You can now accurately say that the volumetric pump will take 3 hours and 20 minutes to infuse Rosie's chemotherapy medication and she can book her transportation home.

If the result is in decimal format, then multiply the decimal by 60, again because there are 60 minutes in one hour. Multiplying a decimal was covered earlier in this chapter should you wish to review it.

To convert a time decimal to minutes, multiply the decimal by 60. Since there are 60 minutes in one hour this will give the exact number of minutes equal to the decimal.

$0.6 \times 60 = 36.0$ minutes

So the number of hours and minutes will be 2 hours 36 minutes. To convert the total time to minutes you could multiply the whole number by 60.

$2.6 \times 60 = 156.0$ minutes

Activity 2.8

Convert the following fractions of hours to a number of minutes.

1. $\dfrac{4}{6}$ 2. $\dfrac{3}{2}$ 3. $\dfrac{3}{5}$ 4. $\dfrac{4}{15}$

5. $\dfrac{7}{6}$ 6. $\dfrac{4}{10}$ 7. $\dfrac{15}{20}$ 8. $\dfrac{4}{5}$

Convert the following hours, shown as decimals, to a total number of minutes.

1. 0.55   2. 3.3   3. 3.1   4. 0.25
5. 12.2   6. 5.45   7. 5.8   8. 0.3
9. 11.5   10. 4.6   11. 7.2   12. 0.75

Addition and subtraction

Most student nurses take it for granted that they can carry out addition and subtraction. Your patients and colleagues will rely on your ability to carry out these tasks accurately. In Chapter 4 (Fluid balance and maintenance) you will use your addition and subtraction skills to calculate your patient's **fluid balance**. The fluid balance is the amount of fluid the patient is retaining to ensure their hydration levels are sufficient to maintain life.

Addition

Scenario

You are currently calculating the fluid balance for Major Thomas Llandar. Major Llandar has been recorded as having consumed the following liquids: tea 800ml, coffee 550ml, water 600ml and juice 175ml over a 24-hour period. You have to calculate Major Llandar's total fluid intake for the day as part of your daily duties, a NMC professional standard requirement (29(ii)).

In order to find the total amount of fluid, you need to add all the amounts of different fluids consumed. The best-practice method is to list the numbers one above the other. Keeping the digits in alignment allows you to total each column of numbers in turn. Should a column total become double digits, place the first digit at the base of the next column to the left. The second digit goes into the total as part of the answer sought.

$$
\begin{array}{r}
175 \\
600 \\
550 \\
800 \\
1 \\
\hline
2125 \text{ ml}
\end{array}
$$

You can now confidently report on his Fluid Balance Chart that Major Llandar has consumed 2125ml of fluid on this day.

Subtraction

Scenario

*You are currently calculating the fluid balance for Major Thomas Llandar. Major Llandar has been recorded as having consumed 2125ml of liquids on the day being charted. His total **fluid output** was recorded as 1960ml. To complete the chart you must now subtract the output from the input to obtain the fluid balance.*

As for addition, align the digits of the numbers above each other. When a value being subtracted is too large to be subtracted from the digit above it, you will need to 'borrow' from the digit to the left in the top number. This will lower the value you borrow from by 1, as can be seen in the diagram, and increase the digit you are subtracting from by 10. These changes are shown using small digits.

$$
\begin{array}{r}
{}^{1}2\ {}^{10}1\ {}^{1}2\ 5 \\
1\ \ 9\ 6\ 0 \\
\hline
0\ \ 1\ 6\ 5 \text{ml}
\end{array}
$$

The result gives Major Llandar a fluid balance of 165ml for the day on which the figures were recorded.

Hint ... You should always subtract the lesser value number from the greater value number. Should the amount expended (output) be more than the amount consumed (intake), this would indicate a Negative Fluid Balance.

A negative balance should be preceded by the word 'Minus' or clearly marked with the – symbol.

Activity 2.9

The following patients are all under observation. For each patient, find the total fluid intake, the total fluid output, and hence the fluid balance. (None of these questions has a negative result.)

1. Janet Barko consumed the following:
    275ml + 75ml + 250ml + 480ml
    The following amounts were recorded as outputs:
    305ml + 212ml + 375ml + 125ml

2. Eddese Grim consumed the following:
    365ml + 305ml + 250ml + 225ml
    The following amounts were recorded as outputs:
    375ml + 160ml + 185ml + 215ml

3. Ali Barker consumed the following:
    485ml + 350ml + 275ml + 176ml
    The following amounts were recorded as outputs:
    450ml + 365ml + 245ml + 175ml

Chapter summary

Patients rely on nurses to accurately calculate their medications as prescribed. Later in this book we will guide you through that skill. In order to do this as part of your duties you must first be able to master the mathematical skills shown in this chapter. The methods and skills you practise and become proficient at here will enable you to become a mathematically proficient nurse.

This chapter is one of the major building blocks on which your nursing career is built and you should feel comfortable doing all the activities provided. Students are often anxious about the mathematics in use throughout nursing because complete accuracy is essential. This anxiety is misplaced, since with practice and by using this book you will gain confidence and realise the simplicity of the calculations required in nursing. Throughout this book, and indeed throughout your career, you can always refer back to this chapter if you need to refresh your memory.

Answers to the activities

Activity 2.1 (page 17)

1. $\dfrac{375}{550} = \dfrac{15}{22}$ 2. $\dfrac{625}{890} = \dfrac{125}{178}$ 3. $\dfrac{325}{375} = \dfrac{13}{15}$ 4. $\dfrac{64}{96} = \dfrac{2}{3}$ 5. $\dfrac{42}{96} = \dfrac{7}{16}$ 6. $\dfrac{24}{69} = \dfrac{8}{23}$

7. $\dfrac{575}{1275} = \dfrac{23}{51}$ 8. $\dfrac{25}{520} = \dfrac{5}{104}$ 9. $\dfrac{45}{475} = \dfrac{9}{95}$ 10. $\dfrac{54}{181} = \dfrac{54}{181}$ 11. $\dfrac{21}{24} = \dfrac{7}{8}$ 12. $\dfrac{35}{230} = \dfrac{7}{46}$

You can revise your times tables using one of the useful websites listed, or any other appropriate source. The ability to cancel down is a skill every nurse can use to make the calculation of drug doses easier to carry out accurately.

Activity 2.2 (page 18)

Weekly requirement = Daily requirement $\times$ 7

Therefore the patients' requirements for seven days will be as follows.

1. Sebastian Contina for 7 days needs 0.105g
2. Jess Crome for 7 days needs 1.05g
3. Steven Gusty for 7 days needs 0.0742g
4. Helen Reckit for 7 days needs 3.15g
5. Mark Strode for 7 days needs 0.847g
6. Alison Barbara for 7 days needs 0.35g.
7. Falua McTaggart for 7 days needs 1.75g
8. Arthur Dat for 7 days needs 38.5g
9. Iain Burns for 7 days needs 0.525g

Accuracy is what every nurse strives to achieve at all times. The ability to multiply numbers containing a decimal point accurately is essential.

Activity 2.3 (page 20)

The amount of drug weight in 1 millilitre of the syrup mixtures is as follows.

1. 1.6mcg/ml
2. 8.1mg/ml
3. 19.5mcg/ml
4. 0.15g/ml
5. 0.375mg/ml
6. 0.88mg/ml
7. 2.3mcg/ml
8. 1.001g/ml
9. 0.024mg/ml

This activity enables you to practise your division and cancelling down methods, skills which every nurse could use many times in their daily duties.

Activity 2.4 (page 21)

The numbers of doses of medication obtained from the amounts are as follows.

1. $8.1 \div 0.9 = 9$
2. $1.5 \div 0.05 = 30$
3. $0.075 \div 0.0025 = 30$
4. $10 \div 2.5 = 4$
5. $0.325 \div 0.025 = 13$
6. $0.090 \div 0.015 = 6$

Activity 2.5 (page 22)

To convert any fraction to a decimal, you divide the number on the top by the number on the bottom.

1. $\dfrac{13}{4} = 3.25$

2. $\dfrac{10}{8} = 1.25$

3. $\dfrac{22}{4} = 5.5$

4. $\dfrac{7}{4} = 1.75$

5. $\dfrac{15}{4} = 3.75$

6. $\dfrac{26}{4} = 6.5$

7. $\dfrac{17}{8} = 2.125$

8. $\dfrac{34}{8} = 4.25$

9. $\dfrac{17}{4} = 4.25$

10. $\dfrac{12}{5} = 2.4$

11. $\dfrac{21}{10} = 2.1$

12. $\dfrac{27}{5} = 5.4$

Activity 2.6 (page 23)

To convert from a fraction to a decimal, use the decimal digits as the numerator and the number 1 followed by as many zeros as decimal places for the denominator. Then use your skills in cancelling down to obtain the simplest or lowest form.

1. $0.50 = \dfrac{1}{2}$

2. $0.25 = \dfrac{1}{4}$

3. $0.375 = \dfrac{3}{8}$

4. $0.08 = \dfrac{2}{25}$

5. $0.044 = \dfrac{11}{250}$

6. $0.04 = \dfrac{1}{25}$

7. $0.125 = \dfrac{1}{8}$

8. $0.075 = \dfrac{3}{40}$

9. $0.010 = \dfrac{1}{100}$

10. $0.072 = \dfrac{9}{125}$

11. $0.200 = \dfrac{1}{5}$

12. $0.875 = \dfrac{7}{8}$

Activity 2.7 (page 24)

If the decimal is equal to or greater than 0.5 or the fraction equal to or greater than $\frac{1}{2}$, then the whole number is increased to the next whole number.

1. $1.7 \rightarrow 2$

2. $4\frac{19}{35} \rightarrow 5$

3. $11.92 \rightarrow 12$

4. $2\frac{6}{7} \rightarrow 3$

5. $59\frac{5}{8} \rightarrow 60$

6. $49\frac{7}{15} \rightarrow 49$

7. $39.6 \rightarrow 40$

8. $25\frac{3}{5} \rightarrow 26$

9. $28.49 \rightarrow 28$

10. $60.4 \rightarrow 60$

11. $21\frac{8}{10} \rightarrow 22$

12. $63.7 \rightarrow 64$

13. $24\frac{14}{29} \rightarrow 24$

14. $17.18 \rightarrow 17$

15. $9.9 \rightarrow 10$

Activity 2.8 (page 26)

To convert a time fraction to a number of minutes, multiply the fraction by 60.

1. $\dfrac{4}{6} = 40$ 2. $\dfrac{3}{2} = 90$ 3. $\dfrac{3}{5} = 36$ 4. $\dfrac{4}{15} = 16$

5. $\dfrac{7}{6} = 70$ 6. $\dfrac{4}{10} = 24$ 7. $\dfrac{15}{20} = 45$ 8. $\dfrac{4}{5} = 48$

To convert the total time to minutes, multiply the number by 60.

1. $0.55 = 33$ 2. $3.3 = 198$ 3. $3.1 = 186$
4. $0.25 = 15$ 5. $12.2 = 732$ 6. $5.45 = 327$
7. $5.8 = 348$ 8. $0.3 = 18$ 9. $11.5 = 690$
10. $4.6 = 276$ 11. $7.2 = 432$ 12. $0.75 = 45$

Activity 2.9 (page 28)

1. Janet Barko consumed the following:
   275ml + 75ml + 250ml + 480ml = 1080ml
   The following amounts were recorded as outputs:
   305ml + 212ml + 375ml + 125ml = 1017ml
   1080 − 1017 = A positive balance of 63ml

2. Eddese Grim consumed the following:
   365ml + 305ml + 250ml + 225ml = 1145ml
   The following amounts were recorded as outputs:
   375ml + 160ml + 185ml + 215ml = 935ml
   1145 − 935 = A positive balance of 210ml

3. Ali Barker consumed the following:
   485ml + 350ml + 275ml + 176ml = 1286ml
   The following amounts were recorded as outputs:
   450ml + 365ml + 245ml + 175ml = 1235ml
   1286 − 1235 = A positive balance of 51ml

Useful websites

For free online guides and resources on basic mathematics revision, refer to the following websites.

BBC Bitesize and Skillswise

The BBC Bitesize and Skillswise websites offer many tutorials which could be used to gain more practice at a basic mathematics level.

1. Times tables grid
   www.bbc.co.uk/skillswise/numbers/wholenumbers/multiplication/timestables/factsheet1.shtml

2. Multiplication methods
   www.bbc.co.uk/skillswise/numbers/wholenumbers/multiplication/timestables/factsheet3.shtml

3. Long multiplication and division
   **www.bbc.co.uk/schools/gcsebitesize/maths/number/multiplicationdivisionrev1.
   shtml**

4. Division using repeated subtraction
   **www.bbc.co.uk/skillswise/numbers/wholenumbers/division/written/factsheet3.
   shtml**

5. Rounding
   www.bbc.co.uk/schools/gcsebitesize/maths/number/roundestimaterev2.shtml

6. Addition
   www.bbc.co.uk/schools/ks2bitesize/maths/number/addition/read3.shtml

7. Subtraction
   www.bbc.co.uk/schools/ks2bitesize/maths/number/subtraction/read3.shtml

OpenLearn

8. Numbers, units and arithmetic
   http://labspace.open.ac.uk/course/view.php?id=3434

9. Rounding and estimation
   http://labspace.open.ac.uk/course/view.php?id=3586

**companion
website**

For further activities and other useful material, visit the companion website at
www.sagepub.co.uk/starkings2e

Chapter 3
Quantity conversions for nurses

NMC Standards for Pre-registration Nursing Education

At the end of this chapter you will have covered some of the numerical calculations required for the Essential Skills Clusters by the first and second progression point and for entry to the register.

28(1)   Takes and records accurate measurements of weight, height/length, body mass index and other appropriate measures of nutritional status.

33(1)   Is competent in basic medicine calculations.

33(2)   Is competent in the process of medication-related calculation in nursing field

Chapter aims

By the end of this chapter you should be able to:

- convert a given weight, be it of a drug or a person, into a greater or lesser metric unit of weight;
- convert a liquid measure from litres to millilitres and from millilitres to litres;
- convert a given measurement of length into a lesser or greater metric unit of length;
- multiply any amount by 10, 100, 1000.

Introduction

In this chapter you will find examples of the kind of calculations you will need to make in converting units of metric measurement. Throughout your career as a nurse you will need to convert these measures in order to be able to make calculations before administering medications. The patient's prescription could be listed in milligrams, while the drug available at your placement is listed in grams. Before you can accurately calculate the patient's requirement, you will need to convert either the amount needed or the available stock so that they use the same unit of measure.

Hint ... The ability to covert metric measures is essential in healthcare; without it, the patient may receive an incorrect dose of medication. Inaccuracy could lead to an accidental overdose of the drug. This could be as much as 1000 times too much. The all-too-frequent mistakes reported as tragedies in the news reinforce the need for accuracy in all your calculations.

Your skill in accurately converting metric measurements will be examined in many formats; for example, in a formative test done without the use of a calculator or as part of a larger scenario question. Such a question may involve a patient prescribed a number of different drugs, some of which require their measures of strength to be converted prior to calculation of their dosage.

You may need to convert a patient's weight or height in order to compare it with a standardised body mass index chart to check for indications of obesity. As in all chapters, it is suggested that you do the activities without the aid of a calculator in order to become more proficient.

Practising liquid, weight and length conversions will help you, as the future nurse, develop the skills to become more confident with the conversions needed. This chapter will cover the various best-practice methods for the types of conversions that nurses will encounter and perform during their careers.

In Figure 3.1, units of liquid measurement are shown on the left, and units of weight measurement on the right (there is no relationship between liquid measures and weight, except that 1ml of water weighs 1g).

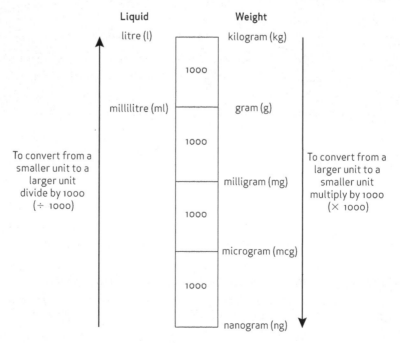

Figure 3.1: Weights and liquids ladder of conversion

Notice that the abbreviation for litre is the small letter l; be careful not to confuse this with the numeral 1.

If you look at the top of the ladder you will see that the largest unit of weight is a kilogram (kg) and the largest commonly used unit for liquids is a litre (l).

The kilogram can be divided up into 1000 units, each of which is known as a gram (g). The gram can then be divided into 1000 units, each being called a milligram (mg). The milligram can then be divided into 1000 units, each of which is a microgram (mcg). Those studying children's nursing will also need to know that the microgram is also divisible into 1000 units, each of which is known as a nanogram (ng). The nanogram is generally seen only in conjunction with children's medical requirements because of the very small size of the metric unit of weight involved. Chapter 7 (Calculations and children) covers smaller dosages in more detail. Great care should be taken not to confuse similar abbreviations when using abbreviations of measurements. See page 2 for more details.

Each litre can be divided into 1000 parts, each of which is called a millilitre (ml). This is as low as a litre is currently divided in most nursing and healthcare situations.

The distance between each rung on the ladder in Figure 3.1 is 1000 units. So we can say there is a 'factor of 1000' between the metric units most commonly used for liquid and weight measures by nurses. The easiest way to handle conversions between these units is to use this fact and simply multiply or divide by 1000, as shown in Figure 3.1 and in the Activities that follow.

Metric units of length are converted differently, and are discussed later in the chapter.

Calculating from one unit to another

Look again at Figure 3.1. On each side of the ladder are instructions about converting between units using either multiplication or division. For example, if you want to convert millilitres to litres, the arrow shows that you have to divide by 1000.

An easy way to do this is to move the decimal point. The number of times the decimal point moves is dictated by the number of zeros in the factor. In the number 1000 there are three zeros, so the point must move three places.

The arrows on either side of the ladder in Figure 3.1 are there to help you remember in which direction to move the decimal point. To convert liquid and weight measures you will always use a factor of 1000, so all you need to decide is whether to move the decimal point to the left or right. Suppose you are required to convert down, from a larger unit to a smaller unit (such as from kilograms to grams); this conversion moves *down* the ladder, and the down arrow is on the *right*. This reminds you to move the decimal point three places to the right.

Multiplying by 1000

You can convert units using this method whether you are changing litres to millilitres or milligrams to micrograms. If the unit you wish to convert from appears above the unit you wish to convert to in the ladder of conversion, then you need to multiply by 1000. You will move the decimal point three places to the *right*; hence the arrow to remind you is on the *right* of the ladder.

Dividing by 1000

There may be times during your training and later in your career where you are called upon to convert a measure upwards. It could be that a patient's fluid balance is being recorded on their chart. Their drink container is marked in millilitres but the information is to be recorded in litres on the chart. In this scenario you would need to go *up* the ladder and the up arrow is on the *left*. The decimal point must go *left* as you need to divide the amount you have in millilitres to obtain the measurement in litres.

For both multiplication and division by 1000, the decimal point will move three places from its original position.

Should a number have no decimal point, then you would start from behind the last digit. In the number 75 there is currently no decimal point showing. However, you can write in the decimal point directly after the last digit, and add some zeros in readiness for conversion, giving, for example, 75.00. If a number already has a decimal point, you should always start your conversion from there; if there are not enough digits to complete the process, you can always add zeros to the front or back of a number before starting to move the decimal point. This will ensure you have no empty spaces when the conversion is completed.

So far we have been multiplying and dividing by 1000. Later in the chapter you will need to multiply or divide by 10 and 100. The number 10 has one zero and so requires a move of just one place, and 100 has two zeros and so the decimal point will move two places: to the left for division or to the right for multiplication.

Scenario

Anne Payne suffers from gastroesophageal reflux disease and has been ordered 20mg of omeprazole to be given orally. As Anne's nurse you have checked the medication available on the ward (stock on hand) and found that the dispensed dose is 0.04g per tablet. Before you can calculate how many tablets Anne will need to take (covered in Chapter 5, Drug calculations), you must convert the units of either the stock on hand (currently in grams) or the ordered amount (currently in milligrams) so that they are both in the same units.

You need to change the units in 0.04g (the stock tablets) to milligrams (mg), to match the units used for the prescribed amount. Converting to the smaller unit will eliminate the decimal point. Putting both the stock required (need) and the stock on hand (have) in the same units means that when you cancel down, as seen in Chapter 2, the 'need' and 'have' unit measures of the drug calculation will cancel each other, leaving just the stock unit measure for your dosage.

$$\frac{\text{Need } \cancel{mg}}{\text{Have } \cancel{mg}} \times \frac{\text{Stock (Unit Measure)}}{1}$$

Let's use Figure 3.1 to do the conversion. Since milligrams (mg) lie below grams (g) on the ladder, then the conversion is to be done using the down arrow, which is on the right, meaning that we have to move the decimal point to the right. So we start with 0.04 and move the decimal point three places to the right:

0 0 4 0. 0

Notice that there were insufficient zeros at the end of the number to complete the conversion, and so two extra zeros have been added.

You now know that the omeprazole tablets on hand are of strength 40.0mg and can accurately calculate the number of tablets required. The last zero and the decimal point can be deleted as they serve no purpose; the tablets are 40mg strength.

Scenario

William Whales has ulcerative colitis and has been ordered 0.75mg of mesalamine to be given orally. Stock on hand is 250mcg capsules. You need to find the strength of mesalamine capsules that William should be given in mcg.

Since micrograms (mcg) lie below milligrams (mg) on the ladder (Figure 3.1), the conversion will be done using the down arrow, which is on the right, so you need to move the decimal point to the right.

0 7 5 0. 0

Again, as there were insufficient places into which to move the point, an extra two zeros were added to 0.75 before the conversion was completed. It is now clear that the amount of mesalamine ordered for Mr Whales is 750.0mcg. Again, the final zero and the decimal point can now be deleted, so the answer is 750mcg.

Now try the following activities to see if you understand how to use the method used in the scenarios to calculate a conversion. You need to make a conversion so that both stock strength (what you *have*) and stock required (what you *need*) are in the same units. You should try the activities without the aid of a calculator.

Activity 3.1

Commonly used as an anticoagulant, warfarin helps to prevent clots in veins, arteries, the lungs or heart. At the Bluebell Care and Respite Centre it is kept in the medicine cabinet in stock strength 5mg, 3mg and 1mg tablets. Patients under your care are being treated with this drug and will be taking their medication daily. At the start of your shift you need to calculate the number of milligrams required for the following patients.

1. Jean Constantine needs to have 0.0250g
2. Michael Crompton needs to have 0.015g
3. Herman Gustov needs to have 0.125g

There are many treatments for hypertension, one of which is the drug prazosin. At the Daffodil Rehabilitation Clinic the following clients are being treated with this drug and will be taking their dosage once a day. The clinical supervisor has tasked you with calculating the number of milligrams required for the following clients.

4. Michaela Burnham needs to have 800mcg
5. Marci Stroud needs to have 0.01g
6. Alistair Mohamed needs to have 5250mcg
7. Abdula Mohamed needs to have 01.25g
8. Sean Payne needs to have 750mcg
9. Ian Reckond needs to have 0.0175g

Answers to all activities can be found at the end of the chapter.

Converting dosages involving mixtures

In the previous section you learned how to convert units of weight for tablets or capsules. In this section we will look at the conversion of drug weights found in medications comprising mixtures and syrups.

Scenario

Fernando, a patient under your care on Tulip Cancer Ward, has been prescribed panitumumab 75mg to slow the growth of his cancer cells. The dispensed dose available on the ward is in a liquid mixture containing 0.1g of drug per 5ml, expressed as 0.1g/5ml. As Fernando's nurse, you need to work out how many milligrams there are in each 5ml in order to allow correct calculation of the dosage to be given to Fernando.

To find out how many milligrams of drug there are in 5ml of a mixture with a strength of 0.1g/5ml you will need to refer back to Figure 3.1. You will need to add extra zeros to the number to provide places for the decimal point to move to. According to the ladder, converting grams to milligrams is *down*, so move the decimal point to the *right*.

The strength in milligram per 5ml mixture is:

0 1 0 0.

You have to move the decimal point three places right as indicated by the ladder. The pani-tumumab strength is 100mg per 5ml, expressed as 100mg/5ml.

The ladder shown in Figure 3.1 can be used to convert metric units of measure for any drug, whatever form it comes in.

Hint . . . A general best-practice rule is to always convert to the smaller unit when dealing with two different weight measures.

If you have to deal with both grams and milligrams, then convert both to milligrams as in the scenario above.

Remember that in a liquid mixture or syrup, only the weight component requires conversion as the liquid volume will always remain the same figure as given.

Activity 3.2

1. Jane is under your care and has been ordered 0.75g of penicillin orally. What is the required amount of penicillin in milligrams for Jane's dose?
2. Mark has been prescribed flucloxacillin. The stock suspension is 1.25g/5ml. What is the stock strength of the medication in mg/5ml?
3. Alison has a mild infection and has been ordered benzyl penicillin from an available mixture of 0.25g/ml. What is this strength in mg/ml?
4. Petula has been ordered paracetamol, and the stock syrup on hand is 0.5g/5ml. What is this strength in mg/5ml?

Activity 3.3

Sertraline is an antidepressant, one of a group of drugs called selective serotonin reuptake inhibitors (SSRIs). Your current placement sees you working in a mental health outpatient clinic and as part of their treatment several service users have been prescribed sertraline to ease their symptoms.

Calculate the following amounts in milligrams for these service users.

1. Diana Johns is prescribed a dose of 0.105g.
2. Joseph Nagel is prescribed a dose of 0.02g.
3. Mary Bengal is prescribed a dose of 500mcg.

continued . . . •••

Pethidine is an analgesic used to ease pain during childbirth. During a placement at a Birthing Centre attached to the regional hospital you are assisting in the care of the following women. They have been prescribed a single dose of pethidine by the Non-Medical Prescribing Nurse in charge at the centre.

Calculate the amount required in micrograms for the following new mothers.

4. Lynne Mohamed is prescribed a dose of 0.25mg.
5. Blessed Masters is prescribed a dose of 0.075mg.
6. Rosalie Jones is prescribed a dose of 0.025mg

A powerful steroidal anti-inflammatory drug in common use is cortisone. During a placement at Willows Retirement and Care Village you will be caring for the following residents, who have mild to severe arthritis and have been prescribed cortisone to ease their pain.

Calculate the amount ordered in milligrams for the following residents.

7. Agatha Hella is prescribed a dose of 750mcg.
8. Hama Aliban is prescribed a dose of 0.03g.
9. Charlotte Burns is prescribed a dose of 0.45g.

Conversion of body weight

At times drug doses may be ordered based on a patient's body weight; this is often the case with children's doses and will be covered in further detail in Chapter 7. Drugs could be ordered in micrograms, milligrams or grams per kilogram per day, which may then be divided up into a number of single doses. So if your patient's personal chart has their weight recorded in grams, you will need to convert this amount to kilograms prior to commencing any calculations for their medication.

Scenario

Eunice Armstrong has been prescribed erythromycin. The dosage prescribed is 4mg/kg/day, four doses daily. Eunice was weighed on Poppet Ward today and recorded at 26500g. Before you can determine the correct dosage Eunice requires, you must convert her recorded weight to kilograms. This will then allow the calculations to be done (as shown in Chapter 5, Drug calculations and Chapter 7, Calculations and children).

To find out how much Eunice weighs in kilograms you again refer to the ladder in Figure 3.1. The weight is in grams and is required in kilograms, which necessitates going up the ladder, and therefore dividing by 1000. Therefore you need to move the decimal point three places to the left.

$$26.5\ 0\ 0$$

So Eunice weighs 26.5kg; as the final zeros have no bearing on the number, they can be deleted. From this information it is now possible to calculate the amount of erythromycin Eunice requires.

Activity 3.4

To help treat infection, particularly after an operation, chloramphenicol is at times given to patients. The following patients on Hibiscus Ward have been ordered chloramphenicol and individual doses will be calculated according to the patient's body weight. Express the following patients' weights in kilograms.

1. Di Goldstein weighs 85070g
2. Roberta Abra weighs 60500g
3. Jess Roberts weighs 26400g
4. Leon Bourke weighs 3050g
5. Lydia Musgrove weighs 965g

Express the following patients' weights in grams.

6. Joe Swift weighs 4.065kg
7. Christo Wrench weighs 0.87kg
8. Lindsey King weighs 41.23kg
9. Dom Oakley weighs 15.75kg
10. Patrice Ngomo weighs 0.635kg

Conversion of metric units in length

The basic metric unit of length is the metre which, like all other metric units, can be divided into smaller units such as the centimetre and millimetre.

The units of length most often used by nurses are metres and centimetres. A metre can be divided into 100 parts, each of which is a centimetre. A metre can also be divided into 1000 parts, with each part known as a millimetre. The millimetre is also equivalent to one-tenth of a centimetre. As with the metric measures used for liquid and weight, the easiest way to illustrate the relationship between metric length measures is with a ladder, as shown in Figure 3.2.

Scenario

*Eunice Armstrong has arrived on the Poppet Ward and as part of the admission process her height was measured at 1.02m. You have been asked to convert her height into centimetres. This height, along with her previously taken weight measure, will then be used on the Body Mass Index and Growth charts currently being used by the **paediatric** department to chart her development.*

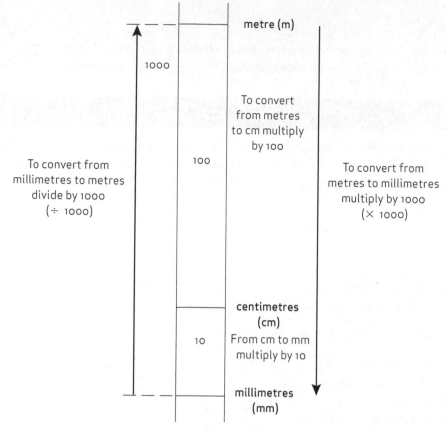

Figure 3.2: Conversion of length in metric units

In the nursing environment you could come across metric length measures in any of the three units shown in the table.

Converting metres to centimetres

To find out how tall Eunice is in centimetres refer to Figure 3.2. Given a height in metres and requiring it in centimetres means you have to move down the ladder, multiplying by 100. As seen in previous conversion activities, multiplying moves the decimal point to the right. Unlike weight and liquid conversions, where a factor of 1000 was universal, here the factor is 100, so you move the point by only two places.

> Hint ... Move the decimal point three places for the factor 1000, which has three zeros, only two places for the factor 100 as it has only two zeros, and only one place for 10 as it has only one zero.

1.02m expressed in centimetres is 102cm.

Converting centimetres to millimetres

If any length given in centimetres is required in millimetres, such as for use on a growth chart, you can again use the ladder for the conversion. The direction is down, as before, but this time only by a factor of 10. The conversion involves moving the decimal point one place to the right, as 10 has only one zero.

$$1\ 02\ 0.\ 0$$

In this example, there were insufficient digits in the number to complete the conversion so extra zeros were added to 102. The result is that 102cm is equal to 1020mm.

Converting metres to millimetres

The use of growth charts is extensive in children's nursing and some of these charts will require length measures in millimetres. You can use the ladder (Figure 3.2) to convert Eunice's height directly from metres to millimetres; the factor is 1000. The conversion therefore involves moving the decimal point three places to the right, as 1000 has three zeros.

$$1\ 0\ \ 2\ 0.\ 0$$

This confirms that Eunice's height in millimetres is 1020mm.

> ### Scenario
>
> *Nadia Gambon on Tulip Ward had her height measured at 1035mm. As an exercise, you have been asked to convert it from millimetres to both centimetres and metres.*

Converting from millimetres to metres

To convert Nadia's height, given in millimetres, to metres, you need to use the ladder in Figure 3.2, this time going upwards. Converting from a smaller to a larger unit requires you to divide. To convert millimetres to metres, the factor is 1000, so you move the decimal point three places to the left.

$$1\ ·0\ \ 3\ \ 5$$

So Nadia's height expressed in metres is 1.035m.

Converting from millimetres to centimetres

To convert from millimetres to centimetres, the factor is 10, so you move the decimal point one place to the left.

$$1\ 0\ 3\ ·\ 5$$

So Nadia's height expressed in centimetres is 103.5cm.

Converting from centimetres to metres

If you need to express a measurement in centimetres as metres, you will need to divide by 100 (because there are 100cm in 1m).

103.5m converts to 1.035m

Activity 3.5

The patients on Tulip Ward have all had their heights measured. As an exercise, you have been asked to convert their heights as follows.

Express the heights of these patients in centimetres.

1. David Brabhim is 1502mm
2. Robin Fosse is 1.35m
3. Aecidia Olin is 1365mm
4. Charles Broome is 1.489m
5. Lata Mouse is 954mm

Convert the units given in the heights of these patients, as indicated.

6. Josephine Swiftly 0.75m, in cm
7. Christian Ferns 0.837m, in cm
8. Lindy Konig 1.38m, in mm
9. Carl Johns 1.09m, in cm
10. Patrice Nomo 1.005m, in mm

Chapter summary

Accurate conversion is an essential skill that every nurse should acquire during their training. This chapter has covered the elements of conversion of metric measures commonly found in healthcare.

In Chapter 5 (Drug calculations) you will see the conversions you have practised here in Chapter 3 put to use when calculating the dosage of medication for patients and service users. You will also come across conversions in Chapter 6 (Calculating intravenous rates) as some intravenous fluids may require conversion of their units of measurement from litres to millilitres before the rate can be calculated. The amount to be given intravenously must be in millilitres to enable the correct calculation.

Answers to the activities

Activity 3.1 (page 38)

Tablets in the Bluebell Centre ward medicine cabinet are of strength 5mg, 3mg and 1mg per tablet.

1. The strength required is 0.0250g.

     So the required amount for Jean Constantine is 25mg.

2. The strength required is 0.015g

     So the required amount for Michael Crompton will be 15mg.

3. The strength required is 0.125g.

     So the required amount for Herman Gustov will be 125mg.

4. The amount required to be converted to mg is 800mcg.

     So the required amount for Michaela Burnham will be 0.8mg. Notice that in this conversion the requirement was to divide, therefore the decimal point moved left. Since no decimal point was shown in the original number, the conversion was started from the right-hand end of the number.

5. The amount required to be converted to mg is 0.01g.

     So the required amount for Marci Stroud will be 10mg.

6. The amount required to be converted to mg is 5250mcg.

     So the required amount for Alistair Mohamed will be 5.25mg. Again in this conversion the requirement was to divide, therefore the decimal point moved left. As no decimal point was shown in the original number the conversion was started from the right-hand end of the number.

7. The amount required to be converted to mg is 1.25g.

     So the required amount for Abdula Mohamed will be 1250mg.

8. The amount required to be converted to mg is 750mcg.

     So the required amount for Sean Payne will be 0.75mg. Notice that in this conversion the requirement was to divide, therefore the decimal went left. Since it was not shown in the original number, the conversion was started from the right-hand end of the number.

9. The amount required to be converted to mg is 0.0175g.

     So the required amount for Ian Reckond will be 17.5mg.

Activity 3.2 (page 39)

1. Jane has been ordered 0.75g of penicillin, so the required amount of penicillin in mg is 750mg.
2. Mark has been prescribed flucloxacillin. On hand is 1.25g/5 ml, so the stock strength in mg/5ml is 1250mg/5ml.
3. Alison was ordered benzyl penicillin 0.25g. The amount required in mg is 250mg.
4. Petula has been ordered paracetamol from the stock syrup of 0.5g/5ml, so the required stock strength is 500mg/5ml of paracetamol.

Refer back to the ladder and the scenario if you are in any doubt about how to carry out the required conversions.

Activity 3.3 (page 39)

1. Diana is prescribed a dose of 0.105g, equal to 105mg
2. Joseph is prescribed a dose of 0.02g, equal to 20mg
3. Mary is prescribed a dose of 500mcg, equal to 0.5mg
4. Lynne is prescribed a dose of 0.25mg, equal to 250mcg
5. Blessed is prescribed a dose of 0.075mg, equal to 75mcg
6. Rosalie is prescribed a dose of 0.025mg, equal to 25mcg
7. Agatha is prescribed a dose of 750mcg, equal to 0.75mg
8. Hama is prescribed a dose of 0.03g, equal to 30mg
9. Charlotte is prescribed a dose of 0.45g, equal to 450mg

Refer back to the ladder and the scenario if you are in any doubt about how to carry out the required conversions.

Activity 3.4 (page 41)

Convert the patients' weights in grams to kilograms.

1. Di Goldstein weighs 85070g ÷ 1000 = 85.07kg
2. Roberta Abra weighs 60500g ÷ 1000 = 60.5kg
3. Jess Roberts weighs 26400g ÷ 1000 = 26.4kg
4. Leon Bourke weighs 3050g ÷ 1000 = 3.05kg
5. Lydia Musgrove weighs 965g ÷ 1000 = 0.965kg

Convert the patients' weights in kilograms to grams.

6. Joe Swift weighs 4.065kg × 1000 = 4065g
7. Christo Wrench weighs 0.87kg × 1000 = 870g
8. Lindsey King weighs 41.23kg × 1000 = 41230g
9. Dom Oakley weighs 15.75kg × 1000 = 15750g
10. Patrice Ngomo weighs 0.635kg × 1000 = 635g

Refer back to the ladder and the scenario if you are in any doubt about how to carry out the required conversions.

Activity 3.5 (page 44)

Convert the patient's height in millimetres or metres to centimetres.

1. David Brabhim is 1502mm ÷ 10 = 150.2cm
2. Robin Fosse is 1.35m × 100 = 135cm
3. Aecidia Olin is 1365mm ÷ 10 = 136.5cm
4. Charles Broome 1.489m × 100 = 148.9cm
5. Lata Mouse 954mm ÷ 10 = 95.4cm

Convert the patients' height in metres to the required unit.

  6. Josephine Swiftly is 0.75m × 100 = 75cm
  7. Christian Ferns is 0.837m × 100 = 83.7cm
  8. Lindy Konig is 1.38m × 1000 = 1380mm
  9. Carl Johns is 1.09m × 100 = 109cm
10. Patrice Nomo is 1.005m × 1000 = 1005mm

Refer back to the ladder and the scenario if you are in any doubt about how to carry out the required conversions.

Useful websites

The following website is useful for metric conversion practice and is free for six months if you register. Try a free download first and register when you need to.

1.   Metric conversions quiz
     www.testandcalc.com/quiz/testmet.htm

     These free websites offer guides and resources on metric measure conversions.

BBC Bitesize

2.   Measures
     www.bbc.co.uk/schools/ks2bitesize/maths/shape_space/measures/read1.shtml

OpenLearn

3.   Numbers, units and arithmetic
     http://labspace.open.ac.uk/course/view.php?id=3434

4.   Rounding and estimation
     http://labspace.open.ac.uk/course/view.php?id=3586

For further activities and other useful material, visit the companion website at
www.sagepub.co.uk/starkings2e

Chapter 4
Fluid balance and maintenance

Chapter aims

By the end of this chapter you should be able to:

*   record fluid intake;
*   record fluid output;
*   complete a Fluid Balance Chart;
*   provide a fluid balance for a 24-hour period.

Introduction

The following case study highlights why it is important to make sure fluid balance calculations are correct.

Case study

Mr Matthews is a patient with bronchitis and his doctor is concerned about how much fluid he takes during the day. A nurse is managing his condition and monitoring his fluid balance. Throughout the day the nurse and Health Care Assistant (HCA) keep a record of the fluids consumed by Mr Matthews (such as water, tea, coffee or juice) and all the fluids he excretes (such as urine and vomit). At 12 p.m. the nurse is chatting to the HCA and makes an error in her reading of Mr Matthews' fluid intake. She records that he drank 50ml of water instead of 500ml of water.

Assuming no further errors took place, Mr Matthews' total recorded fluid intake would be 450ml less than he actually consumed. His total fluid balance would therefore be incorrect and the doctor may be further concerned over the amount of fluid Mr Matthews is taking; he could prescribe extra fluid via an intravenous drip which may not otherwise have been prescribed. So it is important that a patient's fluid is collected and recorded correctly; otherwise a patient may be given extra fluid when it is not required, or given medication to excrete more. Correct fluid balance recording enables the best possible decision to be made by healthcare professionals regarding a patient's well-being and recovery schedule.

Errors made in recording fluid intake and output, and incomplete charts, can have serious consequences for the patient. This chapter goes through the essentials required to complete a Fluid Balance Chart accurately.

A Fluid Balance Chart monitors a patient's fluid status and it is an ESC requirement for this to be completed accurately. As the case above shows, the consequences of not completing the chart accurately can be serious, and so it is an essential skill that needs to be carried out without errors.

Monitoring fluid balance is an essential aspect of nursing and to be effective it should be accurate, otherwise a patient's condition will be assessed on false information. Fluid intake is usually by oral drinks, food, tube feeds and intravenous fluids. Fluid output usually occurs via urine, vomiting, tube drainage, diarrhoea, sweat, gastric secretions or wound drainage. Accurate measurement of a patient's fluid intake and output will identify those patients at risk of becoming dehydrated (lack of fluid) or overhydrated (too much fluid).

This chapter will help you to understand how to calculate fluid balance and fill out a Fluid Balance Chart correctly. We will first look at what a Fluid Balance Chart is and how to calculate fluid balance. We then show you how to work out fluid intake and fluid output. Finally, we will look at entering, interpreting and calculating data on a Fluid Balance Chart. You should use this in conjunction with other resources and training on how to manage fluids, since this book only covers the numeracy requirements for fluid management.

Fluid Balance Charts and calculating fluid balance

A Fluid Balance Chart measurers a patient's hourly fluid intake and output over a 24-hour period. At the end of the 24-hour period the total output (such as urine, drains or other fluid output) is subtracted from the total measured intake (such as oral fluids, intravenous fluids or other inputs). The difference between the input and output is called a fluid balance. It is estimated that an adult person requires between two and a half and three litres of fluid per day.

Fluid balance = Total input − Total output

Alan's fluid balance equals his total intake (or input) of 1738ml minus his total output of 1520ml.

Fluid balance = Total input − Total output
= 1738 − 1520
= 218ml

So the answer is 218ml.

Often the Fluid Balance Chart will not give you the total intake and output but will show you the sums for each intake and output the patient has had. So you need to work out the total intake and output before you can work out the fluid balance.

The scenario below describes what you might face in a practice environment.

Calculating fluid intake

To find the total input, add together all the amounts for the 24-hour period. In this case:

Total input = 250 + 200 + 250 + 300 + 300 + 250 + 300 + 300 + 300
= 2450ml

As you can see, this is an addition calculation, but you need to get this right in order to have the first part of the data needed to calculate the patient's fluid balance.

Calculating fluid output

Once again, to find the patient's fluid output for the 24-hour period, add together all the amounts for the 24-hour period. In this case:

$$\text{Total output} = 300 + 250 + 150 + 300 + 210 + 170 + 200 + 250 + 210 + 200 + 150$$
$$= 2390\text{ml}$$

The fluid balance for Michael Bland is found by subtracting the total output from the total input.

$$\text{Fluid balance} = \text{Total input} - \text{Total output}$$
$$= 2450 - 2390$$
$$= 60\text{ml}$$

In this patient's case the total fluid balance at the end of the 24-hour period is 60ml. Since this is a positive number, it indicates that the patient's intake of fluid is 60ml more than was outputted. However, certain output fluids, such as diarrhoea, are not easy to measure accurately, and it is not possible to measure others, such as sweat. Thus a normal healthy person will appear to have a positive fluid balance. A negative value would indicate that they have excreted more fluid than they have taken in, and that they may become dehydrated.

Now try the following activities to see if you have understood fluid intake and output calculations. You should try the activities without using a calculator.

Activity 4.1

1. Thomas Grain had been given the following fluids during a 24-hour period.

Time	Type	Amount
0600	Tea	200ml
0830	Water	300ml
1030	Juice	300ml
1200	Tea	350ml
1430	Water	200ml
1630	Tea	250ml
1800	Coffee	250ml
1930	Water	150ml
2200	Tea	250ml

    What is Thomas Grain's fluid input for the 24-hour period?

2. Linda Ball's fluid output over 24 hours is measured as follows.

Time	Type	Amount
0600	Urine	300ml
0800	Urine	250ml
0900	Urine	200ml
1030	Urine	300ml
1130	Urine	230ml
1300	Urine	190ml
1500	Urine	250ml
1630	Urine	250ml
1815	Vomit	120ml
1930	Vomit	150ml
2200	Urine	300ml

    What is Linda Ball's output for the 24 hours?

3. Lesley Pain's total intake for a 24-hour period is 2310ml and his total output is 2130ml. What is his fluid balance for the 24-hour period?

Answers to all the activities can be found at the end of the chapter.

The next section shows a typical Fluid Balance Chart and will build on the calculations you have done in Activity 4.1.

Reading, interpreting and completing Fluid Balance Charts

The first section of this chapter should have helped you to become competent in calculating fluid inputs, outputs and balances. The following case study shows how a nurse might use these calculations in a practice setting, using a real Fluid Balance Chart. See if you can understand and follow Vera's observations and conclusions.

Case study

Mr Norman Payne has had a heart attack and is on Daffodil Ward in the Woodland Hospital. Close monitoring of his fluid intake and output is required, using a Fluid Balance Chart (FBC), as in Figure 4.1 on page 55.

Vera, the nurse in charge of Mr Payne, examines his chart and from it she observes:

1. *the time the FBC commenced;*
2. *how much had drained from the tube by 1600;*
3. *what occurred at 1300 hours according to Mr Payne's FBC;*
4. *Mr Payne's fluid balance at the end of the 24-hour period.*

These are her conclusions.

1. *The FBC commenced at 0800 hours. The first line started with 250ml of tea under the intake column.*
2. *By 1600 hours a total of 1200ml had drained from the tube. This is found by adding all the tube drainage, including the 1600 hours line, i.e. 300 + 350 + 200 + 350 = 1200ml.*
3. *At 1300 hours Mr Payne voided 350ml of urine. This is found by reading across from 1300 to find 350ml in the urine column.*
4. *Mr Payne's fluid balance at the end of the 24-hour period is 50ml. This is found by subtracting the total output of urine and tube (total output is 1600 + 350 = 1950) from the total input of 2000. Hence 2000 − 1950 = 50ml.*

Now you have seen how a nurse might use a balance chart, have a go at using one yourself by completing the following activity.

Activity 4.2

Mrs Amelia Blur has pneumonia and is on Tulip Ward in the Woodland Hospital. Her NHS number is NB 01 23 45 C and her date of birth is 21 December 1951. She requires close monitoring of her fluid intake and output using a Fluid Balance Chart.

Mrs Blur was given the following fluids during one 24-hour period:

Time	Type	Amount
0700	Tea	250ml
0900	Water	300ml
1100	Coffee	300ml
1200	Tea	250ml
1500	Water	250ml

continued . . .

1600	Water	300ml
1800	Tea	250ml
1900	Water	200ml
2100	Water	200ml

Mrs Blur's fluid output during the same 24-hour period was measured as follows:

Time	*Type*	*Amount*
0600	Urine	250ml
0700	Urine	200ml
0900	Urine	250ml
1000	Urine	200ml
1100	Urine	200ml
1300	Urine	180ml
1500	Urine	220ml
1600	Urine	150ml
1800	Vomit	120ml
1900	Vomit	100ml
2100	Urine	300ml

Complete a FBC for her, using the practice FBC at the end of the chapter (page 65), and then answer the following questions:

1. What time did the FBC commence?
2. How much in millilitres did Mrs Blur vomit?
3. What occurred at 1100 hours according to Mrs Blur's FBC and what was the fluid balance at this time?
4. What is Mrs Blur's fluid balance at the end of the 24-hour period?

Now you have completed a Fluid Balance Chart, you will realise that is important not only that you get the totals and fluid balance correct, but also that you understand what they mean. So take care in your arithmetic and also try to understand the data and what information this is telling you. Is the patient overhydrated or dehydrated? Do you need to raise any concerns to others on the ward?

It may be useful to look at the fluid charts while you are on placement and ask a member of staff to show you how they are completed, as wards or departments do sometimes complete them differently. For example, some fluid charts document 'insensible loss' (sweat) and this has to be included in the calculation. It is also important that you understand what the words on the fluid chart mean so, again, ask if you need help and check if you are unsure.

Woodland Hospital	Clinical Skills Fluid Balance Chart
Ward: Daffodil	Date: 15/12/10 M/F: M
Family Name: Payne	First Name: Norman
NHS Number: NA 34 56 78 X	Date of Birth: 02/09/32

	INTAKE				OUTPUT				
Time	By Mouth or Tube	ml	Intravenous	ml	Urine ml	Vomit or Tube	ml	Other	ml
0100									
0200									
0300									
0400									
0500									
0600									
0700									
0800	Tea	250							
0900						Tube	300		
1000	Coffee	300							
1100						Tube	350		
1200	Juice	250							
1300					350				
1400	Tea	250				Tube	200		
1500									
1600	Tea	250				Tube	350		
1700									
1800	Coffee	300							
1900						Tube	300		
2000	Coffee	300							
2100	Water	100							
2200						Tube	100		
2300									
2400									
Totals		2000			350		1600		
Total Input	2000				**Total Output**	1950			

Fluid Balance for time period = 2000 − 1950 = 50ml

Figure 4.1: Norman Payne's FBC

Case study

Ms Bisi Blanket has been admitted to Daisy Ward in the Woodland Hospital and has an intravenous drip inserted; 125ml per hour is to be infused. She is not to be given anything orally. Figure 4.2 shows her Fluid Balance Chart.

Natalie, the nurse in charge of Ms Blanket, examines her chart and from it she observes:

continued . . .

1. the FBC commenced at 0300 hours;
2. by 1600 hours 570ml had drained from the tube;
3. by 1100 hours a total of 1125ml had been infused ('infused' here means 'given'; for example, Ms Blanket has received or been given 1125ml of fluid by a drip);
4. at 1700 hours Ms Blanket voided 200ml of urine;
5. the total amount infused is 2000ml;
6. the total output is 770ml;
7. the fluid balance is 1230ml.

Ms Blanket's fluid output may be considered quite low at the moment so you may need to keep monitoring her fluid balance for another 24-hour period, especially considering she has been on an intravenous drip. Intravenous drip rates will be covered in Chapter 6.

Activity 4.3

Look at Mr Omar Mohamed's FBC, shown in Figure 4.3, and answer the following questions.

1. At what time did Mr Mohamed's FBC commence?
   A 0600 hours
   B 0500 hours
   C 1600 hours
2. What occurred at 1500 hours, according to Mr Mohamed's FBC?
   A Mr Mohamed voided 300ml of urine
   B Mr Mohamed was given 250ml of fluid orally
   C Mr Mohamed voided 200ml of urine
3. How much was drained by tube by 1500 hours?
   A 250ml
   B 1000ml
   C 700ml
   D 1250ml
4. How much IV fluid had Mr Mohamed had up to 1100 hours?
   A 100ml
   B 1000ml
   C 700ml
   D 750ml
5. What was Mr Mohamed's fluid balance?
   A 1750ml
   B 2150ml
   C 400ml
   D −400ml

Woodland Hospital

Ward: Daisy

Family Name: Blanket

NHS Number: XY 45 67 89 A

Clinical Skills Fluid Balance Chart

Date: 11/12/10   M/F: F

First Name: Bisi

Date of Birth: 2/12/70

| Time | INTAKE | | | | OUTPUT | | | | |
	By Mouth or Tube	ml	Intravenous	ml	Urine ml	Vomit or Tube	ml	Other	ml
0100									
0200									
0300	Nil orally		Saline	125					
0400				125					
0500				125					
0600				125					
0700				125		Tube	200		
0800				125					
0900				125					
1000				125					
1100				125					
1200				125		Tube	180		
1300				125					
1400				125					
1500				125					
1600				125		Tube	190		
1700				125	200				
1800				125					
1900									
2000									
2100									
2200									
2300									
2400									
Totals					200		570		
Total Input				2000	**Total Output**		770		
Fluid Balance for time period = 2000 − 770 = 1230ml									

Figure 4.2: Bisi Blanket's FBC

Did you find some of these activities more difficult than others? Did you notice, for example, that the question in part 3 was asking how much was drained by tube, not how much was outputted altogether by 1500 hours? You need to take care to understand what is being asked, or what information you need to find out, and ensure you read the chart correctly and find the appropriate data before beginning the calculation. This skill is essential for a registered nurse and will be important from the very start of your practice placements.

Woodland Hospital

Ward: Bluebell

Family Name: Mohamed

NHS Number: CD 56 78 90 B

Clinical Skills Fluid Balance Chart

Date: 09/10/10   M/F: M

First Name: Omar

Date of Birth: 6/03/21

| Time | INTAKE | | | | OUTPUT | | | | |
	By Mouth or Tube	ml	Intravenous	ml	Urine ml	Vomit or Tube	ml	Other	ml
0100									
0200									
0300									
0400									
0500	Nil orally		Saline	100					
0600				100		Tube	300		
0700				100					
0800				100		Tube	350		
0900				100					
1000				100					
1100				100		Vomit	250		
1200				100					
1300				100		Tube	350		
1400				100					
1500					300				
1600	Water	250							
1700					200				
1800	Tea	300							
1900					200				
2000	Water	100							
2100									
2200	Water	100			200				
2300									
2400									
Totals		750		1000	900		1250		
Total Input		1750			**Total Output**		2150		

Fluid Balance for time period = 1750 − 2150 = −400ml

Figure 4.3: Omar Mohamed's FBC

Children's fluid balance

Children's fluid balance is calculated in the same way as the adult ones you have been looking at. The major difference is that a child's fluid intake and output will usually be much lower than that of an adult. You will also have to calculate, particularly for very young children, how much urine has been outputted from a wet nappy.

To find how much urine Omar has passed, you need to subtract the weight of the dry nappy from the weight of the wet nappy. You need to remember 1g = 1ml. So the amount of urine passed in this case is $127 - 15 = 112$ ml.

The 112ml is then added under the urine column of Omar's FBC at the time you weighed the nappy and will be used to calculate his total fluid output and, in turn, his fluid balance.

Activity 4.4

Grace Adoma-Boateng is 8 weeks old and has been admitted to hospital. She has a wet nappy. The nappy weighed 20g when dry, and her nappy now weighs 114g. How much urine did Grace pass since her last nappy change?

Case study

Miss Amber Brown has been admitted to Buttercup Ward in the Woodland Hospital with respiratory problems. She has been put on close monitoring of her fluid intake and output using a Fluid Balance Chart (see Figure 4.4).

Julie, the nurse looking after Amber, has found that a nappy change at 2300 hours was not recorded. Her fluid balance will now have to be altered to include the urine passed at this time. Her dry nappy would have weighed 25g. Her wet nappy weighed 164g.

First we calculate the amount of urine passed: $164 - 25 = 139$ml. This amount is then added to her fluid output giving a total fluid output of $737 + 139 = 876$ml. Her fluid balance will now be $749 - 876 = -127$ml. This value indicates that she has excreted more fluid than she has taken in over this time period. Since this is a negative value it would be wise to pass this information on to the health official in charge of Amber's case.

This is an example of a child's FBC. Now have a go at the following activity.

Woodland Hospital

Ward: Buttercup

Family Name: Brown

NHS Number: 654321

Clinical Skills Fluid Balance Chart

Date: 02/05/10   M/F: F

First Name: Amber

Date of Birth: 21/01/10

Time	INTAKE				OUTPUT					
	By Mouth or Tube	ml	Intravenous	ml	Urine ml	Vomit or Tube	ml	Other	ml
0100									
0200									
0300									
0400									
0500									
0600	SMA Milk	150			155				
0700									
0800									
0900									
1000	SMA Milk	127			143				
1100									
1200					125				
1300									
1400	SMA Milk	172			100				
1500									
1600									
1700									
1800	SMA Milk	125			154				
1900									
2000									
2100					60				
2200	SMA Milk	175							
2300									
2400									
Totals									
Total Input	749				**Total Output**	737			

Fluid Balance for time period = 749 − 737 = 12ml

Figure 4.4: Amber Brown's FBC

Activity 4.5

Master Hadi Ahmad has been admitted to Buttercup Ward in the Woodland Hospital with suspected Swine Flu. He has been put on close monitoring of his fluid intake and output using a Fluid Balance Chart. All dry nappies for Hadi weigh 25g. His NHS number is 765432 and his date of birth is 28 March 2010. Complete a FBC for him, using the practice chart at the end of the chapter.

continued . . .

1. Hadi's nappy was changed at the following times:

Time	*Weight* (g)
0500	175
0930	132
1300	154
1715	143
2100	168

    Add the amount of urine passed to Hadi's Fluid Balance Chart.

2. Hadi was given feeds of SMA Milk:

Time	*Amount* (ml)
0530	130
0915	125
1230	120
1700	122
2130	100

    Add these to Hadi's Fluid Balance Chart.

3. Now work out Hadi's fluid balance.

Chapter summary

Accurate recording of fluid intake and output is a requirement for nurses. Do remember to measure all fluid intake and output and record the amount, along with the type of fluid. If you delegate the task, make sure you get the correct totals. For example, if a patient is able they could record their own intake and output using appropriate measuring devices. Measure all fluids, as far as possible, in a calibrated container so that measures are accurate. Update the FBC on a regular basis. The fluid balance for a 24-hour period is calculated by using the following formula:

Fluid balance = Total input – Total output

Answers to the activities

Activity 4.1 (page 52)

1. Total input = 200 + 300 + 300 + 350 + 200 + 250 + 250 + 150 + 250 = 2250ml
2. Total output = 300 + 250 + 200 + 300 + 230 + 190 + 250 + 250 + 120 + 150 + 300 = 2540ml
3. Fluid balance = Total input − Total output
    = 2310 − 2130
    = 180ml

If you got the arithmetic incorrect here you may wish to refer to Chapter 2 on addition and subtraction, and/or look at web pages 1, 2 and 3, listed at the end of this chapter, for further practice.

Activity 4.2 (page 53)

The FBC below shows how you should have filled in the chart.

Woodland Hospital	Clinical Skills Fluid Balance Chart
Ward: Tulip	Date: 11/06/10 M/F: F
Family Name: Blur	First Name: Amelia
NHS Number: NB 01 23 45 C	Date of Birth: 21/12/51

| Time | INTAKE | | | | OUTPUT | | | | |
	By Mouth or Tube	ml	Intravenous	ml	Urine ml	Vomit or Tube	ml	Other	ml
0100									
0200									
0300									
0400									
0500									
0600					250				
0700	Tea	250			200				
0800									
0900	Water	300			250				
1000					200				
1100	Coffee	300			200				
1200	Tea	250							
1300					180				
1400									
1500	Water	250			220				
1600	Water	300			150				
1700									
1800	Tea	250				Vomit	120		
1900	Water	200				Vomit	100		
2000									
2100	Water	200			300				
2200									
2300									
2400									
Totals	2300				1950		220		
Total Input	2300				**Total Output**		2170		
Fluid Balance for time period = 2300 − 2170 = 130ml									

Figure 4.5: Amelia Blur's FBC

1. The Fluid Balance Chart commenced at 0600 hours.
2. Mrs Blur vomited 120ml at 1800 hours and 100ml at 1900 hours. Her total vomit is therefore 120 + 100 = 220ml.
3. Mrs Blur had 300ml of coffee and voided 200ml of urine. Mrs Blur's total input at 1100 hours is 250 + 300 + 300 = 850ml and her total output is 250 + 200 + 250 + 200 + 200 = 1100ml. Her fluid balance is then total input − total output which is 850 − 1100 = −250ml. Hence her fluid balance at 1100 hours is −250ml.
4. Mrs Blur's fluid balance is 130ml.

Activity 4.3 (page 56)

1. B
2. A
3. B
4. C
5. D

Activity 4.4 (page 59)

The amount of urine passed by Grace is 114 − 20 = 94ml.

The 94ml is then added under the urine column of Grace's FBC at the time you weighed the nappy and will be used to calculate her total fluid output and, in turn, her fluid balance.

Activity 4.5 (pages 60–1)

The FBC shows how you should have filled in the chart.

Remember to take off the weight of the dry nappy, in this case 25g, from the weight of the wet nappy to get the correct urine total. The amount of urine at 0500 hours is then 175 − 25 = 150ml. The correct urine totals to be placed on the FBC are as follows:

Time	Weight (g)	Urine (ml)
0500	175	150
0930	132	107
1300	154	129
1715	143	118
2100	168	143

Fluid balance = Total input − Total output
= 597 − 647
= −50ml

Hadi's fluid balance is −50ml

	Woodland Hospital					Clinical Skills Fluid Balance Chart				
	Ward: Buttercup					Date: 03/05/10 M/F: M				
	Family Name: Ahmad					First Name: Hadi				
	NHS Number: 765432					Date of Birth: 28/03/10				

	INTAKE					OUTPUT				
Time	By Mouth or Tube	ml	Intravenous	ml	Urine ml	Vomit or Tube	ml	Other	ml	
0100										
0200										
0300										
0400										
0500					150					
0600	SMA Milk	130								
0700										
0800										
0900										
1000	SMA Milk	125			107					
1100										
1200										
1300	SMA Milk	120			129					
1400										
1500										
1600										
1700	SMA Milk	122								
1800					118					
1900										
2000										
2100					143					
2200	SMA Milk	100								
2300										
2400										
Totals										
Total Input		597			Total Output		647			
Fluid Balance for time period = 597 − 647 = −50ml										

Figure 4.6: Hadi Ahmad's FBC

Useful websites

The following websites offer revision material that you can use to enhance your numeracy skills. The pages listed below are accessible free of charge and can be used to help you with the arithmetic required for this chapter.

BBC Bitesize

1. Addition
    www.bbc.co.uk/schools/ks2bitesize/maths/number/addition/read1.shtml

2. Subtraction
    www.bbc.co.uk/schools/ks2bitesize/maths/number/subtraction/read1.shtml

Mathcentre

3. Rules of arithmetic
    www.mathcentre.ac.uk/students.php/health/arithmetic/rules/resources/

Appendix

Sample FBC

Woodland Hospital	Clinical Skills Fluid Balance Chart
Ward:	Date: M/F:
Family Name:	First Name:
NHS Number:	Date of Birth:

	INTAKE				OUTPUT				
Time	By Mouth or Tube	ml	Intravenous	ml	Urine ml	Vomit or Tube	ml	Other	ml
0100									
0200									
0300									
0400									
0500									
0600									
0700									
0800									
0900									
1000									
1100									
1200									
1300									
1400									
1500									
1600									
1700									
1800									
1900									
2000									
2100									
2200									
2300									
2400									
Totals									
Total Input					**Total Output**				

For further activities and other useful material, visit the companion website at
www.sagepub.co.uk/starkings2e

Chapter 5
Drug calculations

Chapter aims

By the end of this chapter you should be able to:

- calculate the number of tablets required for patients from their prescription;
- calculate the dose required in liquid form as prescribed;
- calculate the drug dose for injection;
- calculate the drug dose for injection for patients requiring insulin;
- work out the dose to be given to a patient when prescribed by body weight.

Introduction

The following case study highlights why it is important to make sure drug calculations are correct.

> ### Case study
>
> *Susan's nursing duties include giving the pre-medication for patients about to have surgery in the operating theatre; this relaxes the patient before they are wheeled down to the theatre. The anaesthetist can then place an endotracheal tube into the patient's trachea in order to ensure that the airway is not closed off and that air can reach the lungs during surgery.*
>
> *An inexperienced doctor drew up what he thought was the correct pre-medication dose for one of Susan's patients, but made a mistake in the volume required and underestimated the dose. The result was that the patient was not sufficiently relaxed and was extremely uncomfortable when the endotracheal tube was inserted.*
>
> *The endotracheal tube can be inserted in an emergency without the aid of any relaxation but this is extremely uncomfortable and generally to be avoided in other circumstances. In some cases the anaesthetist is unable to insert the endotracheal tube and surgery has to be postponed, causing distress to patients and disturbance to schedules.*
>
> *Correct calculations are essential for all concerned.*

This chapter covers a variety of numerical and mathematical tasks which nurses may be required to perform in practice.

This book does not cover reconstitution of a powder drug. Drugs are mainly stored in powder form because they are often unstable in liquid form and are only made up into a solution just before use. Consult the pharmacist at your place of work for help in reconstitution of solutions.

During your nursing career you will administer and later supervise the administration of all types of medicines. To do this safely the development of certain numerical and mathematical skills, as seen in Chapter 2, is essential. Your calculations must be accurate in order to ensure that the safety of patients is not compromised.

During your course your ability in drug calculations will be examined, usually by a series of tests which help you develop your skills and which are done without the use of a calculator. This is to check that you have mastered the ESC 33(i) and 33(ii). It is suggested that you practise the calculations in this chapter without using a calculator. If your training institution allows you to use one then by all means do so, but be aware that some assessments may need to be completed without using a calculator.

Many nurses have difficulty with drug calculations, usually because they are not confident with the numeracy and mathematics required. Practising drug calculations will help you develop these skills and become more confident with the calculations needed. Checking colleagues' calculations is another way to check your understanding of the numerical concepts involved in drug calculations.

Many drugs require some type of calculation prior to administration, and before you start this chapter you will need to be able to convert from one metric unit to another. Chapter 3 has examples of this skill and can be used for revision if necessary. Table 5.1 is a reminder of the types of conversions with which you will need to be familiar.

Unit	Abbreviation	Equivalent	Abbreviation
1 kilogram	kg	1000 grams	g
1 gram	g	1000 milligrams	mg
1 milligram	mg	1000 micrograms	mcg
1 microgram	mcg	1000 nanograms	ng
1 litre	l	1000 millilitres	ml

Table 5.1: Equivalents of common units of measurement

Notice that the abbreviation for litres is the small letter 'l': be careful not to confuse this with the numeral 1.

How drugs are administered

There are three main ways that drugs can be administered:

*   **orally** (by mouth);
*   by **injection**;
*   or by **intravenous infusion**.

This chapter will look at drugs given orally by tablets or in liquid form and by injection. Intravenous infusion will be covered in Chapter 6. You will need to apply previous knowledge in order to complete this chapter so look back, particularly at Chapters 2 and 3, and revise when you need to.

Calculating a dose involving tablets

Drugs may be administered in many ways; a common means is orally, in the form of tablets. Whole tablets are always preferable to broken tablets; never use less than half a tablet for a patient. Broken tablets are harder to identify as many tablets look the same and a patient could be given the wrong tablet, which will not help their recovery progress. If a tablet has been broken in half always use the 'other' half for the next dose for the same patient, making sure you keep the broken tablet in the correctly labelled container. Tablets are often marked with the weight of drug which they contain.

Figure 5.1: Oral medications

As with any calculation involving the administration of drugs, it is absolutely vital that the same unit of weight is used throughout the calculation. Weight is the amount of drug contained in the tablet. Always check that both the **prescribed strength** (what is required by the patient) and the **stock strength/dispensed dose** (the weight of tablet in the medicine cabinet) are in the same units. For example, both could be in milligrams (mg), or both in micrograms (mcg).

Often one of the units needs to be converted and this must be done before any calculation is started (Chapter 3 covers conversion rates). This ensures that the patient gets the correct dose. For example, if the prescribed dose is in milligrams and the tablets are in micrograms, ignoring the units would mean that the patient could be given an incorrect dose. An incorrect calculation of this sort can seriously harm a patient's recovery or indeed cause further illness.

It is safer, and therefore best practice, to convert to the lowest level of unit. Once the strength required and stock strength are both in the same units, we can calculate the number of tablets required.

The method for calculating the number of tablets is the same for all drug doses, and uses this formula:

$$\frac{\text{Strength required}}{\text{Stock strength}} \times \text{Volume of stock solution}$$

Since we are dealing with tablets here, the volume of the stock solution will always be one tablet. Therefore the formula for calculating how many tablets a patient should receive is:

$$\frac{\text{Strength required}}{\text{Stock strength}} \times \text{One tablet}$$

Since tablets are never broken to less than half a tablet, the answer should always be half a tablet, a whole number of tablets, or a whole number plus half a tablet. However, bear in mind that if the tablet is not scored (with a groove down the middle) it must not be broken and the dose given must be to the nearest tablet.

Check with the patient's consultant and/or pharmacist if you have any concern about the dose. For example, if you think the dose is too high or low for the patient, then it is always best to check.

You may find it helpful to use this mnemonic:

N = Need (the **strength required/prescribed strength**)
H = Have (what you have as **stock strength**)
S = Stock (volume of **stock strength**)

And the formula in this case would be

$$\frac{N}{H} \times \frac{S}{1} = \text{The correct dose for the patient}$$

The numeral 1 under the 'S' is there to prevent you making mistakes during your calculations.

> ## Scenario
>
> *Ethel Orchison suffers from epilepsy and has been ordered 45mg of phenobarbitone to be given orally. Stock on hand is 30mg tablets. You need to find the number of tablets required for Ethel.*

To find out how many tablets Ethel requires, you need to abstract the relevant pieces of information. The strength required here is 45mg and the stock strength is 30mg. Using the formula above and inserting the relevant values we do the calculation:

$$\frac{\text{Strength required}}{\text{Stock strength}} \times \text{One tablet}$$

$$\frac{45}{30} \times 1 = 1\frac{1}{2} \text{ tablets}$$

Or, using the NHS mnemonic where you Need 45mg, you Have 30mg, and the Stock is one tablet:

$$\frac{N}{H} \times \frac{S}{1} = \text{The correct dose for the patient}$$

$$\frac{45}{30} \times 1 = 1\frac{1}{2} \text{ tablets}$$

So Ethel needs to take $1\frac{1}{2}$ tablets to get 45mg of phenobarbitone as prescribed. (Please note although this example has half a tablet for illustrative purposes, you should check in your own practice whether breaking a tablet is allowable.)

Notice that both the stock strength and the strength required are in milligrams, so no conversion between units is necessary. The next scenario is one where a conversion has to take place before the formula can be used.

> ## Scenario
>
> *Thomas Bailey has heart problems and has been ordered 0.25mg of digoxin to be given orally. Stock on hand is 125mcg tablets. You need to find the number of tablets that Thomas should be given.*

Notice that the stock required (what you need) is in milligrams (mg) and the stock strength (what you have) is in micrograms (mcg). First you need to convert these both to the same units. Using Table 5.1 we can see that to get 0.25mg into micrograms we move the decimal point (equivalent to multiplying by 1000) three places to the right as follows:

0.25mg = 250mcg

Now both stock strength (Have) and strength required (Need) are in the same units and we can use the formula above to put in the numerical values.

$$\frac{\text{Strength required}}{\text{Stock strength}} \times \text{One tablet}$$

$$\frac{250}{125} \times 1 = 2 \text{ tablets}$$

Or, using the NHS mnemonic where you Need 250mg, you Have 125mg, and the Stock is one tablet we have:

$$\frac{N}{H} \times \frac{S}{1} = \text{The correct dose for the patient}$$

$$\frac{250}{125} \times \frac{1}{1} = 2 \text{ tablets}$$

So Thomas needs to have two tablets of digoxin from the stock cupboard to get the correct dose as ordered.

Now try the following activities to see if you have understood how to use the formula to calculate how many tablets the patients require. Remember that you may need to do a conversion so that both stock strength (what you have) and stock required (what you need) are in the same units. You should try the activities without using a calculator.

Activity 5.1

Warfarin is an anticoagulant and helps to prevent clots in veins, arteries, lungs or heart. Warfarin comes in tablet form; the tablets that are kept in the medicine cabinet are of stock strength 5mg; they are scored. The following residents at Garden View care home are being treated with this drug and will be taking the tablet(s) once a day. Calculate the number of tablets required for the following patients.

1. Simon Estra needs to have 12.5mg
2. Jerry Connors needs to have 7.5mg
3. Steven d'Guy needs to have 0.005g

Prazosin is an antihypertensive drug which works by relaxing the blood vessels. The stock strength of the tablets kept in the medicine cabinet is 2mg per tablet; the tablets are scored. The following patients with high blood pressure are being treated with this drug once a day. Calculate the number required for the following patients.

4. Hesta Forram needs to have 6mg
5. Marc McWords needs to have 0.002g
6. Jai Mohamed needs to have 5mg

continued . . .

Thioridazine is in a class of drugs called phenothiazines. The drug works by changing the actions of chemicals in the brain and is typically used for psychotic disorders, such as schizophrenia. Thioridazine is generally reserved for people who do not respond to other drugs or who cannot take other drugs because of their side effects. The strength of stock kept in the medicine cabinet is 50mg per tablet; the tablets are scored. The following patients are being treated with this drug in one daily dose. Calculate the number of tablets required for the following patients.

7. Fatima Patel needs to have 0.1g
8. Susanna Payne needs to have 75mg
9. Ian Whitless needs to have 0.05g

Answers to all the activities can be found at the end of the chapter.

The questions in Activity 5.1 refer to tablets and not capsules. If drugs are in capsule form, then you must not open or split them. Doses are calculated to the nearest whole capsule. Should you have any queries, consult the person in charge at your place of work and/or the pharmacist or doctor who prescribed the drug.

Some drugs come in various forms such as mixtures, capsules or even powder, which is mixed with water before the drug is given. You must take great care when reading the prescribed order regarding in what form the drug is to be given. The next section will look at drugs in liquid form.

Calculating a dose involving mixtures

Drugs are often stocked in the form of suspensions, syrup or mixtures. Before measuring out any of these mixtures you should thoroughly shake the container so that the drug is evenly mixed, otherwise the incorrect dose may be given.

Having ensured that the mixture is thoroughly mixed, you can measure the prescribed dose. To calculate the amount required, use the same method as for all drug calculations, with this formula:

$$\frac{\text{Strength required}}{\text{Stock strength}} \times \text{Volume of stock solution}$$

Alternatively, use the NHS mnemonic:

$$\frac{N}{H} \times \frac{S}{1} = \text{The correct dose for the patient}$$

Scenario

Lenny Mitchell, from Bluebell Children's Home, has been ordered three doses of 500mg of penicillin per day to treat his bacterial infection; stock mixture on hand is syrup 125mg/5ml. You need to work out what volume of syrup per dose should be given to Lenny, and his total daily dose.

To find out how many millilitres Lenny requires you need to abstract the relevant pieces of information. The strength or amount required is 500mg and the stock strength is 125mg/5ml. The 125mg/5ml means that there is 125mg of drug per 5ml of mixture.

Using the formula or NHS mnemonic above gives the following calculation:

The volume required, in ml, is $\dfrac{500}{125} \times \dfrac{5}{1}$.

First you cancel down, as shown in Chapter 2. Cancel by 125, since 125 goes once into 125 and four times into 500, giving:

$$\frac{4}{1} \times \frac{5}{1} = 4 \times 5 = 20\text{ml}.$$

So Lenny needs 20ml of the mixture to receive 500mg of penicillin as prescribed per dose. His total dose for the day (he is to be given three doses) is then found by multiplying the dose by three, that is, $20 \times 3 = 60$ml.

This prescription has both the stock strength and the strength required in milligrams so no conversion was required. The next scenario is one where a conversion has to take place before the formula can be used.

Scenario

Larry, a patient on Daisy Ward, has been ordered flucloxacillin 0.4g orally to treat his chest infection; stock syrup on hand is 125mg/5ml. You need to work out what volume of syrup should be given to Larry.

Notice here that the units are different; one is in grams and the other is in milligrams. You need to convert the prescribed dose to milligrams before you use the formula. Refer to Table 5.1 on p68 for conversion rates. In this case 0.4g = 400mg (you move the decimal point three places to the right).

The strength or amount required is 400mg and the stock strength is 125mg/5ml.

Using the formula or NHS mnemonic given above gives the following calculation:

The volume required, in ml, is $\dfrac{400}{125} \times \dfrac{5}{1}$.

First you cancel down, as shown in Chapter 2. Cancel by 25, since 25 goes 5 times into 125 and 16 times into 400, giving

$$\frac{16}{5} \times \frac{5}{1}.$$

You can then cancel out the 5s to give 16ml. So Larry needs 16ml of the mixture to receive 400mg of flucloxacillin as prescribed.

Whether the drug is in the form of a syrup or in a suspension, the calculation remains the same; in both cases, always shake the container to ensure a proper distribution of the drug before measuring.

Remember, before doing any calculations make sure that the strength required and stock strength are in the same units. As a general rule of thumb, always convert to the smaller unit; for example, if you are dealing with both grams and milligrams, it is better to work in milligrams, as in the scenario with Larry above.

You should try the following activities without using a calculator. Answers to the activities can be found at the end of the chapter.

Activity 5.2

1. Jane from Bluebell Respite Centre has been ordered 0.75g orally of penicillin for her throat infection; stock syrup on hand is 250mg/5ml. What volume of syrup is required for her dose?
2. Max, a mental health service user, has a severe chest infection and has been prescribed 0.5g flucloxacillin orally; stock suspension on hand is 125mg/2.5 ml. How much stock suspension is required per dose for him? He is to have four doses per day. How much flucloxacillin does he receive in one day?
3. Alison has a wound infection after her operation and has been ordered benzyl penicillin 700mg orally; stock mixture on hand is 250mg/5ml. Calculate the volume of mixture to be given to Alison.
4. Tricia has been ordered paracetamol 150mg three times a day orally to help ease her pain after having her wisdom teeth out; stock syrup on hand is 125mg/5ml. What volume of syrup should be given to Tricia per dose? How much paracetamol does she receive per day?

So far we have looked at drugs that have been given orally. The next two sections will look at drugs that are administered by injection.

Calculating a drug dose for injection

The previous section looked at drugs in liquid form that were given orally; another way of administering drugs in liquid form is by injection. When calculating a dose to be given by injection the number of decimal places used in the calculations should match the graduations on the syringe that you are going to use (see Figures 5.3 and 5.4 below).

Notice that, unlike tablets where the dose is calculated in whole and half numbers, liquids to be given by injection can be measured in a narrower range.

As with any calculation involving the administration of drugs, it is absolutely vital that the same unit of capacity is used throughout the calculation. Always check that both strength required and stock strength are in the same unit. The most common is to have both in grams (g), both in milligrams (mg) or both in micrograms (mcg). Any conversion must be done before the dosage calculation is started. See Chapter 3 for revision on conversions.

The volume that the liquid is prepared in must also be noted, because the result of the calculation will be an amount in this unit of measure. For example, if the drug comes in milligrams per millilitre the required dose will be calculated and drawn up in millilitres (ml). In the case of insulin, which comes in units, then the dose would be drawn up in units.

Once the strength required and stock strength are both in the same units of measurement, you can begin to calculate the amount of stock solution required. The formula for calculating liquid drug doses is the same as for those we have already done:

$$\frac{\text{Strength required}}{\text{Stock strength}} \times \text{ Volume of stock solution}$$

Alternatively, use the NHS mnemonic:

$$\frac{N}{H} \times \frac{S}{1} = \text{ The correct dose for the patient}$$

As well as calculating the correct volume of drug to be given, you also need to select the correct syringe to use and draw up the volume required. Typical sizes of syringes used for injections in hospitals and clinics in the UK are 1ml, 2ml, 3ml, 5ml, 10ml, 20ml, 30ml and 50ml.

Figure 5.2: A typical type of syringe

For example, if you need to draw up 0.8ml then you would use a 1ml syringe (see Figure 5.3).

To draw up 3ml you would use a 3ml syringe (see Figure 5.4).

Figure 5.3   *Figure 5.4*

So first work out, using the formula, how much drug in volume you need to administer; then select the correct syringe size; and finally draw up the volume required.

Scenario

Scopolamine, an anticholinergic medicine, is being used to ease Mrs Vera Bland's nausea as she recovers from surgery. She has been ordered 0.25mg of scopolamine. Stock on hand is 0.4mg/2ml. You need to work out how much is to be drawn up for her dose.

To find out how much is to be drawn up for Vera's injection you need to abstract the relevant pieces of information. Notice that the amount prescribed and the stock on hand are both in decimal form. It is easier if you convert both amounts to micrograms; using the conversion Table 5.1 you have:

0.25mg = 250mcg
0.4mg = 400mcg

The strength required (Need) is 250mcg.
The stock strength (Have) is 400mcg.
The volume of stock solution (Stock) is 2ml.

Using the formula or NHS mnemonic given above gives the following calculation:

$$\frac{\text{Strength required}}{\text{Stock strength}} \times \text{Volume of stock solution}$$

Alternatively, use the NHS mnemonic:

$$\frac{N}{H} \times \frac{S}{1} = \text{The correct dose for the patient}$$

$$\frac{250}{400} \times \frac{2}{1} = 1.25\text{ml}$$

So you need to select a 2ml syringe to draw up the 1.25ml required for Vera's injection (see Figure 5.5).

Figure 5.5

A common error made here is to just ignore (or misread due to haste) the decimal points. This would result in the following calculation:

$$\frac{25}{4} \times \frac{2}{1} = 12.5\text{ml, which is } \textit{incorrect.}$$

This would result in a huge overdose for the patient, as well as a large volume to be injected.

Now try the following activities and see if you can work out how much drug to draw up and what syringe size to use.

Activity 5.3

Morphine is in a group of drugs called narcotic pain relievers. It is used to treat moderate to severe pain. The following patients in Roseland Hospice have cancer and have been prescribed morphine to ease their pain.

Morphine of stock strength 15mg/ml is in the medicine cabinet. Calculate the amount to be drawn up and the syringe size to use for injection for the following patients.

1. Diana Vittel is prescribed a dose of 18mg
2. Jose Mercado is prescribed a dose of 7.5mg
3. Mary Nearly is prescribed a dose of 0.072g

Pethidine is a painkilling drug used to ease pain during labour. The following patients have been prescribed a single dose of pethidine.

The stock strength of pethidine in the medicine cabinet is 100mg/2ml. Calculate the amount to be drawn up and the syringe size to use for injection for the following patients:

4. Linda Myers is prescribed a dose of 70mg
5. Mitac Patel is prescribed a dose of 55mg
6. Rose Mint is prescribed a dose of 0.05g

Cortisone is a powerful anti-inflammatory medication. The following residents in Sunland Farm Care Home have arthritis and have been prescribed cortisone to ease their inflammatory pain.

Cortisone of stock strength 125mg/5ml is in the medicine cabinet. Calculate the amount to be drawn up and the syringe size to use for injection for the following patients.

7. Daniel Agbosi is prescribed a dose of 70mg
8. Hadan Ali is prescribed a dose of 45mg
9. Carolyn Blean is prescribed a dose of 0.05g

The next section will look at giving injections of insulin.

Calculating a drug dose by injection for insulin doses

The strength of insulin is measured by the number of insulin units contained in 1ml. For example U.10 or 10U means that there are 10 units of insulin per millilitre. A 1ml syringe would normally be used. This syringe is graduated in tenths of a millilitre.

Syringes are usually graduated in units for the type of insulin prescribed so make sure you use the correct syringe or you will have to adjust the volume required. Insulin keeps blood glucose levels under control for people with diabetes, and is prescribed in terms of units.

Scenario

John Edwards has U.40 insulin and needs to have a dose of 28 units. You have a syringe graduated to be used with U.40 insulin. You need to work out how much is to be drawn up for him using the U.40 insulin.

U.40 means that there are 40 units contained in one millilitre. You need to find the amount to draw up into the syringe so that John gets a dose of 28 units. This is a fraction problem; you need to find what proportion 28 units is of 40 units. This can be expressed as a fraction:

$$\frac{28}{40} = 0.7\text{ml}$$

John is to have 0.7ml of insulin drawn up for his injection.
Fractions were covered in Chapter 2 so look back if you need to revise here.
Now try the following activities to test your understanding of insulin doses.

Activity 5.4

1. Two patients newly diagnosed with diabetes at the Diabetes Clinic require insulin injections.

Name	Dose to be given	Strength of solution
Paula Blond	20 units	U.20
Juliet Moone	50 units	U.40

    How much insulin is to be drawn up for these patients using the strengths given?

2. A syringe is graduated in units for use with U.40 insulin. To what graduation mark should it be filled to give a dose of 12 units, if only U.20 insulin is available?

We now look at drugs that are prescribed by body weight.

Drug dose by body weight

At times drug doses may be ordered based on a patient's body weight, especially with children's doses (see Chapter 7). When calculating body weight doses you need to make sure that all measurements are in the same units before working out the dose required. For revision on conversions see Chapter 3.

Drugs will usually be ordered in milligrams per kilogram of body weight per day, divided up into a number of doses per day. So first of all calculate the total dose for the day for the patient and then divide up this total into the number of doses per day. Remember that you always need to calculate the single dose rate so as to administer the correct dose each time.

> ### Scenario
>
> *Emma Austen has been prescribed erythromycin. The dose prescribed is 50mg/kg/day, four doses daily. Emma was weighed today, in the care home, and her weight is 84kg. You need to find what total dose Emma requires and then calculate the single dose to be given to her.*

To find out how much Emma requires you need to abstract the relevant pieces of information. The dose 50mg/kg/day means that for every kilogram Emma weighs she needs 50mg of erythromycin; Emma weighs 84kg. So the total daily requirement for Emma is $84 \times 50 = 4200$mg. Emma is to be given four doses a day, so you need to divide the 4200mg into four equal doses.

$4200 \div 4 = 1050$mg per dose.

Emma needs each dose to be of 1050mg.

Now try the following activities regarding dose by body weight. Children's doses will be covered in Chapter 7.

Activity 5.5

Chloramphenicol is given to patients, particularly after an operation, to help treat infection. The following patients, on your ward, have been ordered chloramphenicol by their body weight. Calculate the total dose prescribed and how much each dose in milligrams is to be for the following patients.

1. Dana Gould weighs 63kg and is prescribed 40mg/kg/day to be given in four doses.
2. Roberta Asham weighs 57kg and is prescribed 100mg/kg/day divided into doses to be given every 6 hours for the next 24 hours.
3. Jess Awardo weighs 84kg and is prescribed 50mg/kg/day in three doses.

Calculating drug doses in mental health nursing

People with mental health-related conditions should always be treated in the same way as others in your care and are often known as service users to avoid any of the unjustified stigma historically attached to conditions such as manic depression, bipolar disorder or Tourette's syndrome. As with patients in clinical or surgical wards, their conditions can be managed or alleviated with correct medication.

The following activity allows for the opportunity to experience calculations carried out with the types of medication used in the treatment of people with mental health disorders.

Activity 5.6

1. Your patient Jackson has been ordered olanzapine, an anti-psychotic used for his schizophrenia and bipolar 1 mania. His medication is to be given by intra-muscular injection due to his current mixed episodes associated with bipolar disorder. The consultant has ordered a dose of 7.5mg from your available stock of 5mg/ml. What volume should you draw?

2. Marie has schizophrenia and also endures the effects of Tourette's syndrome. She has been prescribed haloperidol in order to control her condition at a rate of 3mg per dose given 6 times a day. Her medication is available in stock ampoules of 5mg per ml. Given that she will need this medication for her entire respite stay of 3 days, calculate how much is required per dose and for the duration of her visit.

3. Alistair has a major depressive disorder and he has been ordered selegiline transdermal treatment. The effective dosage range is between 6 and 12mg per 24 hours. Alistair's doctor has recommended a dosage of 63mg, given over a period of a week in equal amounts. Calculate the volume of treatment to be given to Alistair daily.

4. Trudi has been ordered donepezil hydrochloride to assist in the treatment of her Alzheimer's disease. She will begin on a dose of 5mg per day for 3 weeks then 10mg for a further 3 weeks before starting on the maximum dosage of 23mg per day. What amount of donepezil hydrochloride will Trudi have had in grams after an initial 12 weeks of treatment?

Chapter summary

Accurate drug calculation is an essential skill that nurses have to acquire during their training, before they can be entered on the professional register for nurses. This chapter has covered the basis for drug calculations for tablets and for drugs in liquid form to be taken *continued . . .* •••

orally or by injection. Doses of insulin and doses by body weight have been introduced; children's drug calculations by body weight will be covered later in Chapter 7.

Always check the prescription drawn up for a patient. If a dose is written in micrograms and the stock supplied is in milligrams you will need to convert milligrams to micrograms in order to calculate the dose required. It is usual to convert to the lowest level of unit. For all drug calculations, make sure that you have both stock strength and stock required in the same unit of measurement.

The next chapter will look at intravenous (IV) drip rates as some drugs are administered via an IV drip.

Answers to the activities

Activity 5.1 (page 71)

For questions 1–3, tablets in the medicine cabinet are of strength 5mg per tablet and the tablets are scored.

1. The strength required is 12.5mg and the stock strength is 5mg.

$$\frac{\text{Strength required}}{\text{Stock strength}} \times \text{ One tablet}$$

$$\frac{12.5}{5} \times 1 = 2\frac{1}{2} \text{ tablets}$$

Or using the NHS mnemonic where you **N**eed 12.5mg and you **H**ave 5mg and the **S**tock is one tablet:

$$\frac{N}{H} \times \frac{S}{1} = \text{ The correct dose for the patient}$$

$$\frac{12.5}{5} \times \frac{1}{1} = 2\frac{1}{2} \text{ tablets}$$

So Simon Estra needs to take $2\frac{1}{2}$ tablets to get 12.5mg of warfarin as required.

Alternatively you could convert both to micrograms to remove the decimal point:

12.5mg = 12500mcg and 5mg = 5000mcg so the formula is $\frac{12500}{5000} \times \frac{1}{1} = 2\frac{1}{2}$ tablets.

2. The strength required here is 7.5mg and the stock strength is 5mg so Jerry Connors needs $\frac{7.5}{5} \times \frac{1}{1} = 1\frac{1}{2}$ tablets.

Alternatively you could convert both to micrograms to remove the decimal point:

7.5mg = 7500mcg and 5mg = 5000mcg so the formula is $\frac{7500}{5000} \times \frac{1}{1} = 2\frac{1}{2}$ tablets.

3. Since the stock strength is 5mg and the stock required is 0.005g we need to convert both to mg before using the formula. See Chapter 3 on how to do conversions if you need some revision here. 0.005g = 5mg so the formula is $\frac{5}{5} \times \frac{1}{1} = 1$ tablet. Steven d'Guy needs 1 tablet.

For questions 4–6, tablets in the medicine cabinet are of strength 2mg per tablet and the tablets are scored.

4. The strength required here is 6mg and the stock strength is 2mg and the formula is $\frac{6}{2} \times \frac{1}{1} = 3$ so Hesta Forram needs 3 tablets.

5. The strength required here is 0.002g and the stock strength is 2mg so we need to convert to mg before using the formula. See Chapter 3 on how to do conversions if you need some revision here. 0.002g = 2mg so the formula is $\frac{2}{2} \times \frac{1}{1} = 1$ so Marc McWords needs 1 tablet.

6. The strength required here is 5mg and the stock strength is 2mg and the formula is $\frac{5}{2} \times \frac{1}{1} = 2\frac{1}{2}$ so Jai Mohamed needs $2\frac{1}{2}$ tablets.

For questions 7–9, tablets in the medicine cabinet are of strength 50mg per tablet and the tablets are scored.

7. The strength required here is 0.1g and the stock strength is 50mg so we need to convert to mg before using the formula. See Chapter 3 on how to do conversions if you need some revision here. 0.1g = 100mg so the formula is $\frac{100}{50} \times \frac{1}{1} = 2$ so Fatima Patel needs 2 tablets.

8. The strength required here is 75mg and the stock strength is 50mg. $\frac{75}{50} \times \frac{1}{1} = 1\frac{1}{2}$ so Susanna Payne needs $1\frac{1}{2}$ tablets.

9. The strength required here is 0.05g and the stock strength is 50mg so we need to convert to mg before using the formula. See Chapter 3 on how to do conversions if you need some revision here. 0.005g = 5mg so the formula is $\frac{50}{50} \times \frac{1}{1} = 1$ so Ian Whitless needs 1 tablet.

If you got the arithmetic incorrect here you may wish to refer back to Chapter 2 on using fractions, or to Chapter 3 on conversions. You could also look at the web pages listed at the end of those chapters for further practice. Remember that you are multiplying, not adding, here; this is a common error that can harm patients, so be careful.

Activity 5.2 (page 74)

1. The stock required and the stock strength are in different units so we first convert them to the same units. 0.75g = 750mg (see Table 5.1 for conversions). The 250mg/5ml means that there is 250mg per 5ml of mixture.

    $$\frac{750}{250} \times \frac{5}{1} = 15\text{ml} \qquad \text{so Jane needs 15ml for her dose.}$$

2. $$\frac{500}{250} \times \frac{2.5}{1} = 10\text{ml} \qquad \text{so Max needs 10ml per dose.}$$

    He has 4 doses per day so his total dosage is $4 \times 10 = 40$ml.

3. $$\frac{700}{250} \times \frac{5}{1} = 14\text{ml} \qquad \text{so Alison needs 14ml per dose.}$$

4. $$\frac{150}{125} \times \frac{5}{1} = 6\text{ml} \qquad \text{so Tricia needs 6ml per dose.}$$

    She has 3 doses per day so her total dosage is $3 \times 6 = 18$ml.

Activity 5.3 (page 77)

For questions 1–3, morphine is of 15mg/ml in the medicine cabinet.

1. The strength required (Need) is 18mg, the stock strength (Have) is 15mg, the volume of stock solution (Stock) is 1ml

    $$\frac{18}{15} \times \frac{1}{1} = 1.2\text{ml}$$

    So you need to select the 2ml syringe to draw up the 1.2ml required for Diana's injection.

2. The strength required is 7.5mg, the stock strength is 15mg and stock volume is 1ml.

    $$\frac{7.5}{15} \times \frac{1}{1} = 0.5\text{ml}$$

    Select the 1ml syringe and draw up 0.5ml of morphine for Jose.

3. The strength required is 0.072g, the stock strength is 15mg and stock volume is 1ml. Notice here that the amount prescribed and the stock on hand are in different units so we need to convert both to milligrams, using Table 5.1.

    $$0.072\text{g} = 72\text{mg}$$

    $$\frac{72}{15} \times \frac{1}{1} = 4.8\text{ml}$$

    So select the 5ml syringe and draw up 4.8ml of morphine for Mary.

For questions 4–6, pethidine is of 100mg/2ml in the medicine cabinet.

4. The strength required is 70mg, the stock strength is 100mg and stock volume is 2ml.

    $$\frac{70}{100} \times \frac{2}{1} = 1.4\text{ml}$$

    So select the 2ml syringe and draw up 1.4ml of pethidine for Linda.

5. The strength required is 55mg, the stock strength is 100mg and stock volume is 2ml.

    $$\frac{55}{100} \times \frac{2}{1} = 1.1\text{ml}$$

    So select the 2ml syringe and draw up 1.1ml of pethidine for Mitac.

6. The strength required is 0.05g, the stock strength is 100mg and stock volume is 2ml.

    Notice here that the amount prescribed and the stock on hand are in different units so you need to convert both to milligrams, using Table 5.1.

    $$\frac{50}{100} \times \frac{2}{1} = 1\text{ml}$$

    So we select the 1ml syringe and draw up 1ml of pethidine for Rose.

For questions 7–9, cortisone is of 125mg/5ml in the medicine cabinet.

7. The strength required is 70mg, the stock strength is 125mg and stock volume is 5ml.

    $$\frac{70}{125} \times \frac{5}{1} = 2.8\text{ml}$$

    So select the 3ml syringe and draw up 2.8ml of cortisone for Daniel.

8. The strength required is 45mg, the stock strength is 125mg and stock volume is 5ml.

    $$\frac{45}{125} \times \frac{5}{1} = 1.8\text{ml}$$

    So select the 2ml syringe and draw up 1.8ml of cortisone for Hadan.

9. The strength required is 0.045g, the stock strength is 125mg and stock volume is 5ml.

    In this case the units are different so you need to convert them both to milligrams, using Table 5.1.

    0.05g = 50mg

    $$\frac{50}{125} \times \frac{5}{1} = 2\text{ml}$$

    So select the 2ml syringe and draw up 2ml of cortisone for Carolyn.

Activity 5.4 (page 78)

1. Paula Blond has been prescribed 20 units. The U.20 contains 20 units per ml strength, so you need that amount drawn up in the syringe.

    1ml = 20 units

    So draw up 1ml of U.20 into the syringe for injection.

    Juliet Moone has been prescribed 50 units. The U.40 contains 40 units per ml.

    1ml = 40 units

    $\frac{1}{4}$ml = 10 units

    So 50 units = $1 + \frac{1}{4} = 1\frac{1}{4}$ml

    $1\frac{1}{4}$ml is the same as 1.25ml so you draw up 1.25ml of the U.40 insulin into the syringe for injection.

    An alternative way of calculating this is:

    40 units = 1ml

    1 unit = $\frac{1}{40}$

    50 units = $\frac{1}{40} \times 50 = 1\frac{1}{4}$ml

    This method will work for all insulin calculations.

2. The syringe is graduated for 40 units. The insulin that is available is U.20.

    To give 12 units of U.40 you need to double the dose.

    $12 \times 2 = 24$ units

Activity 5.5 (page 79)

1. Dana weighs 63kg and is prescribed 40mg per kg in body weight to be given in 4 doses. Her total prescribed is $63 \times 40 = 2520$mg. For each dose you divide the total by 4 (i.e. number of doses per day) so $2520 \div 4 = 630$mg.

2. Roberta weighs 57kg and is prescribed 100mg per kg in body weight per day. Roberta's total dosage is $57 \times 100 = 5700$mg per day. This is to be divided into doses to be given every 6 hours for the next 24 hours. The number of doses will be $24 \div 6 = 4$ doses per 24-hour period. $5700 \div 4 = 1425$mg so each dose is of 1425mg. So Roberta has 4 doses at 6-hour intervals of 1425mg per dose.

    A common mistake made here is to divide the total dose of 5700mg by 6, the interval time between doses, rather than by 4, the number of actual doses. This would give $5700 \div 6 = 950$mg, meaning the patient is given a greatly reduced dosage.

3. Jess weighs 84kg and is prescribed 50mg per kg in body weight per day. Total dosage per day is $84 \times 50 = 4200$mg. This is to be divided into three doses. So each dose is $4200 \div 3 = 1400$mg.

Activity 5.6 (page 80)

Much of the care you give as a mental health nurse may be given in the service user's environment, such as their home or assisted living accommodation. The location should have no bearing on the crucial requirement for total accuracy in your calculations, so although the location is different, the methods used to find the accurate dosage remain the same.

$$\frac{\text{Strength required}}{\text{Stock strength}} \times \text{ Volume of stock solution}$$

Or using the NHS mnemonic:

$$\frac{N}{H} \times \frac{S}{1} = \text{ The correct dose for the service user}$$

1. Using the formula we have

    $$\frac{7.5}{5} \times \frac{1}{1} = 15\text{ml} \qquad \text{So Jackson needs 1.5ml per dose}$$

2. Using the formula we have

    $$\frac{3}{5} \times \frac{1}{1} = 0.6\text{ml}$$

    So Marie needs 0.6ml per dose, given 6 times daily, which means she requires $0.6 \times 6 = 3.6$ml. Since Marie will be staying for 3 days you will need to have $3.6\text{ml} \times 3 = 10.8$ml available during her stay.

    Total medication required for 3 days is 10.8ml.

3. This question gave an amount to be taken by Alistair over the week or 7 days and asks for the daily dosage. You must simply divide the user's prescribed requirement by the length of time for which it has been ordered.

    $63 \div 7 = 9$mg/day is needed by Alistair.

4. Trudi suffers from Alzheimer's and her consultant needs to monitor her total consumption of the drug to ensure guidelines on the maximum dosage are maintained. Your task is to calculate the amount of drug taken in total for 12 weeks, but remember to convert your result to grams before reporting your finding.

    $(5 \times 7 \times 3) + (10 \times 7 \times 3) + (23 \times 7 \times 6) = 1281\text{mg} = 1.281\text{ gram}$

    Did you remember the dosage ordered was the daily amounts for each week?

Useful websites

The following websites offer revision material that you can use to enhance your numeracy skills. If you need to revise any of the skills covered earlier, for example in Chapters 2 and 3, look at the web pages listed at the end of those chapters.

Testandcalc

The following website is useful for drug calculations practice and is free for six months if you register. Try a free download first and register when you need to.

1.   Drug calculations quiz page
     www.testandcalc.com/quiz/index.asp

Nursing Standard

The *Nursing Standard* has online guides and resources that you can use free of charge. The following two, among others, relate to drug calculations.

2.   Improving the numeracy skills of nurse presribers
     http://nursingstandard.rcnpublishing.co.uk/resources/archive/GetArticleById. asp?ArticleId=4534

3.   Drug calculations part 1: a critique of the formula used by nurses
     http://nursingstandard.rcnpublishing.co.uk/resources/archive/GetArticleById. asp?ArticleId=6542

For further activities and other useful material, visit the companion website at **www.sagepub.co.uk/starkings2e**

Chapter 6
Calculating intravenous rates

NMC Standards for Pre-registration Nursing Education

At the end of this chapter you will have covered some of the numerical calculations required for the Essential Skills Clusters by the first and second progression point and for entry to the register.

32(2)   Monitors and assesses people receiving intravenous fluids.
33(1)   Is competent in basic medicines calculations.
33(2)   Is competent in the process of medication-related calculation in nursing field
36(4)   Safely manages drug administration and monitors effects.
38(4)   Safely and effectively administers and where necessary prepares medicines via routes and methods commonly used and maintains accurate records.

Chapter aims

By the end of this chapter you should be able to:

* calculate the flow rate in drops per minute that an intravenous infusion chamber should be set to in order to ensure an accurate delivery flow to individual patients;
* calculate the amount of time required for a volumetric infusion pump to deliver a given volume;
* calculate the flow rate required for a volumetric infusion pump to deliver a volume of fluid in a specified amount of time.

Introduction

These chapter aims may sound a little daunting, but you will soon become familiar with the terms used, and understand the procedures. As a nurse you will need to be able to calculate the rate at which a fluid or medication is to be given to a patient by way of an intravenous infusion (IV). It is a very common form of therapy, as you will see.

Case study

This extract is taken from the Indian Journal of Pharmacology *and shows the importance of correct medication and observation:*

Case study

A 7-month-old girl was referred with a history of high-grade fever for 4 days, lethargy, poor feeding for 2 days, hematochezia and ooze from IV puncture sites. The child was drowsy on examination with poor hemodynamic status, hepatomegaly, and free fluid in the abdomen. During illness she had received 5 doses of 250 mg tablets of paracetamol, that is, 178 mg/kg/day (weight 7 kg) along with 3 doses of 100 mg of mefenamic acid per day (ie, 43 mg/kg/day). She was admitted in the ICU and given supportive therapy. She was given an IV loading dose of NAC. However, within 24 hours, her general condition deteriorated and she succumbed to multiorgan failure.

Some patients need a drug continuously, rather than in separate doses. One way of delivering medicine that way is by intravenous infusion; this is by infusing the drug in a liquid directly into a vein. As a student nurse, you will learn how to set up and calculate intravenous infusion rates.

Intravenous infusion may also be used when a patient is unconscious and so cannot swallow. Some drugs and certainly blood transfusions always need to be delivered directly into the circulatory system. The registered nurse needs to be able to calculate the flow rate and the amount of time for the volume of drug/blood to be given.

Some patients that you see will require IV drugs that are keeping them alive. So errors that might not matter with some patients could be very serious for others. Most errors arise when the nurse makes mistakes in their calculations. It is like driving a car and breaking the speed limit; sometimes there is no adverse outcome, but on some occasions things go wrong and a tragedy occurs. What we can conclude from the report findings is that nurses need to make sure that all drugs administered via an IV are calculated correctly – and this chapter will show you how.

It is not only drugs that you, as a nurse, will assist in administering intravenously. It is very common in hospital to 'give fluids' this way. The fluids could be plasma or blood products needed after a patient loses blood during surgery or trauma such as a road traffic accident. Your patient may require replacement of body fluids lost for a variety of medical reasons, such as in cases of severe burns. Some patients will require an IV because they need to be hydrated, to prevent or lessen potential liver damage following an overdose of acetaminophen, or during a course of chemotherapy. The following scenario is one where fluids given to a child had terrible consequences.

Case study

This story is taken from a South African newspaper and was published in November 2009 (Star, 2009). Celina Kometsi took her two-year-old daughter to her local hospital to be treated for burns on her hands. Two IV drips were inserted into the child's feet containing fluid which was infused for three hours. The child was reported to be in a great deal of pain and her feet started to swell and also turned purple.

A child's condition should always be monitored by a nurse and any problems, especially like the one above, should be reported to the doctor or consultant treating the patient. This story did not have a happy ending as the child had to have both her legs amputated just below the knee. Most IVs that you will be responsible for will not result in this serious condition but it does highlight the need for close monitoring.

In this chapter we will explain how to calculate the IV rate for two types of IV apparatus that are commonly used to give a patient their medication.

- In the first section we explain the calculation required to determine the rate of an IV using a **giving set** with **drip chamber.**
- In the second section you will learn to calculate the rate required using an IV **volumetric pump**.

When using the IV volumetric pump, you will need to be able to calculate the time required to deliver a volume of fluid, given the pump rate in millilitres per hour (ml/h). Activities on delivery rate required given the time to be taken will also feature in this chapter.

When you are tested on these calculations, you may not be allowed to use a calculator, so as you practise them you should attempt them without the aid of a calculator. Current recommendations from the Royal College of Nursing suggest that nursing students do not use calculators in their studies.

In Chapter 3 (Quantity conversions for nurses), you practised how to convert litres to millilitres. If you feel you need to revise this, go back to Chapter 3 and practise. You will need to understand that calculation for the activities in this chapter. Intravenous calculations with a drip chamber set are done with the IV fluid amount in millilitres and so require conversion before calculation.

You may also want to review Chapter 2 (Essential numeracy requirements for nursing), as both cancelling down and the rounding of fractional or decimal values will also be used in this chapter.

Drip chamber giving sets

There are three main types of drip chamber or giving set in use throughout the healthcare system.

- **Macrodrip**: in which the chamber converts each millilitre of fluid into 15 drops; this is generally used for infusion of blood or other blood products such as **platelets** or **plasma**.
- Macrodrip: in which the chamber converts each millilitre of fluid into 20 drops; this is generally used for infusions such as normal saline or 5 per cent dextrose.

The size of the drops is controlled by the fixed diameter of the plastic delivery tube. The drip rate delivered by each particular set is marked on the packaging of the IV giving set, so make sure that you select and use the correct drip size.

- **Microdrip**: in which the chamber converts each millilitre of fluid into 60 drops; this is generally used in critical care situations.

The giving set is the device used to break down the flow of each millilitre of fluid into droplets which can then be counted to ensure the correct number of droplets per minute for each of your patients. You should always ensure that you correctly identify the giving set to be used by *personally checking* its packaging. To correctly calculate the flow rate of the giving set with a drip chamber, follow this simple formula.

$$\text{IV flow rate} = \frac{\text{IV amount in ml} \times \text{giving set}}{\text{Hours} \times 60}$$

Notice that the bottom of the fraction is the time over which the IV is to be given in hours multiplied by 60. This is equivalent to the time in minutes. If the time over which the IV is to be given is already in minutes, you do not need to convert it to hours or multiply it by 60. If the time is given as hours and minutes, convert it to a total number of minutes; you do not need to multiply the result by 60. If you need practice with time conversions, revise Chapter 2.

Scenario

Nicola Burke has had surgery and is now regaining consciousness from the anaesthetic in the recovery ward. As you are on placement in Gerbera Ward you have been tasked to set up an IV for Nicola. The consultant has ordered 1 litre of Lactated Ringer's solution over eight hours using a 20 drops/ml Macrodrip set.

As the amount to be given is in litres, you will first need to convert this to millilitres. Chapter 3 (Quantity conversions for nurses) covers this in detail; revise this calculation if necessary. Having converted the IV amount to millilitres, put all the information into the formula.

$$\text{IV rate} = \frac{1000 \times 20}{8 \times 60}$$

This calculation can be cancelled down as shown in Chapter 2 (Essential numeracy requirements for nursing).

$$\text{IV rate} = \frac{125 \times 1}{1 \times 3} = \frac{125}{3} = 41\tfrac{2}{3} \text{ or } 41.66 \text{ drops/min}$$

As quite often occurs when calculating an IV rate, the numbers do not cancel out to an exact number of drops per minute. No matter how you try it is not usually possible to divide a droplet into a fraction or decimal, hence fractional and decimal answers require rounding. If you need to revise this skill, again refer back to Chapter 2.

The fraction $\tfrac{2}{3}$ or the decimal 0.66 is more than half way to the next whole number and so the answer is rounded up to 42.

The IV for Nicola needs to be set at 42 drops/minute to ensure she receives her prescribed IV over the period of time set.

You should try this chapter's activities without the aid of a calculator.

Activity 6.1

It has been a busy day in the operating theatre, and the following patients have all arrived in the Gerbera Ward recovery room. Calculate the rate of the IV for each of the following patients for the amounts of Hartmann's solution (CSL) listed. Each IV solution will be using a Macrodrip 20 drops/ml drip chamber giving set.

1. Thom Flynn 750ml over 8 hours
2. Francisca Hall 1.3 litre over 9 hours
3. Simon Cramp 1 litre over 5 hours
4. Kareb Mohamed 500ml over 3 hours
5. Poppy Brock 900ml over 5 hours

Calculate the rate of the IV for each of the following patients for the amounts of Lactated Ringer's solution listed. Each IV will be using a Macrodrip 20 drops/ml drip chamber giving set.

6. Jessica Wallace $\frac{3}{4}$ litre over $7\frac{1}{2}$ hours
7. Thomas Major 1.85 litres over a day
8. Meow Felinez 750ml over 5 hours 45 minutes
9. Nassir Hussein $1\frac{1}{4}$ litre over 12 hours
10. Poppy Seedz 3 litres over 24 hours

Answers to all the activities can be found at the end of the chapter.

For the infusion of blood, platelets or plasma, a Macrodrip chamber that converts each millilitre of fluid to be given into 15 drops/ml is most commonly used.

Scenario

*Nazeem Ali has had a traffic accident and requires a blood plasma infusion. You are on placement in the Accident and Emergency Ward and have been tasked to set up the infusion for Nazeem. The **registrar** has ordered 750ml of plasma over 2 hours using a 15 drop/ml Macrodrip set.*

As the amount to be given is in millilitres there is no need to convert before calculating the flow rate. Place the given information directly into the formula.

$$\text{IV flow rate} = \frac{750 \times 15}{2 \times 60}$$

This calculation can be cancelled down as shown in Chapter 2 (Essential numeracy requirements for nursing).

$$\text{IV rate} = \frac{375 \times 1}{1 \times 4} = \frac{375}{4} = 93\frac{3}{4} \text{ or } 93.75 \text{ drops/min}$$

Again, the IV rate does not cancel to an exactly even answer. The fraction $\frac{3}{4}$ or the decimal 0.75 is over half way to the next whole number and so the answer is rounded up to 94. Refer back to Chapter 2 for rounding fractions and decimals if needed.

The infusion for Nazeem needs to be set at 94 drops/min to ensure she receives her prescribed IV over two hours.

Activity 6.2

You are working at a day centre on Sunshine Ward, which cares for patients suffering with haemophilia. The following patients are each to receive a plasma product as part of their treatment. Calculate the IV rate for each of the patients given the amounts of medication listed. Each IV will be delivered using a Macrodrip 15 drops/ml drip chamber giving set.

1. Nigella Faroff 1 litre over 10 hours
2. Wendy Wassit $\frac{1}{2}$ litre over 5 hours
3. Alistair Abdul $\frac{3}{4}$ litre over 6 hours
4. Jodi James 750ml over 5 hours
5. John Johnstone 250ml over 150 minutes

The third type of drip chamber is the Microdrip, which converts each millilitre of fluid into 60 drops. This chamber is commonly found in critical care settings.

Scenario

Heather has been rushed to hospital suffering from an accidental overdose of acetaminophen, a common ingredient of over-the-counter painkillers. After several hours in the Accident and Emergency Department (A&E) Heather has been transferred to the critical care ward. You are required to install a new IV for Heather which delivers 1 litre of acetylcysteine over 16 hours using a Microdrip giving set drip chamber.

As the amount to be given is in litres you will first need to convert this amount to millilitres. Refer to Chapter 3 (Quantity conversions for nurses) for conversion of litres to millilitres if necessary. Having converted the amount to millilitres, put the information directly into the formula.

$$\text{IV flow rate} = \frac{1000 \times 60}{16 \times 60}$$

This calculation can be cancelled down as shown in Chapter 2 (Essential numeracy requirements for nursing).

$$\text{IV rate} = \frac{125 \times 1}{2 \times 1} = \frac{125}{2} = 62\tfrac{1}{2} \text{ or } 62.5 \text{ drops/min}$$

The fraction $\frac{1}{2}$ or the decimal 0.5 is half way to the next whole number and so is rounded up to 63. Refer back to Chapter 2 for rounding of fractions and decimals if necessary.

The IV for Heather needs to be set at 63 drops/minute to ensure she receives the IV amount prescribed over the correct time period.

Activity 6.3

Following a busy period in Woodlands Hospital A&E the following patients have been transferred to the Carnation Critical Care Unit where you are on shift. Calculate the rate of IV infusion for each of the following patients using a Microdrip 60 drops/ml giving set drip chamber for the amounts of IV fluid shown.

1. Ghana Khartoum $\frac{1}{2}$ litre over 5 hours
2. Lucy Freeman 200ml over 75 minutes
3. Linda Peters 0.75 litre over 4 hours
4. Hilda Hammer 500ml over 6 hours
5. Carol Johnstone 0.1 litre over 1 hour

Volumetric IV pump

The other most frequently used method of intravenous infusion is a volumetric pump. The pump is used to deliver rates of fluids at 5ml or more per hour in most nursing applications.

Scenario

Adeoti Khan is to receive 5 per cent dextrose (D5W) over a period of 10 hours following her collapse while running a marathon. The volumetric infusion pump has been set at a rate of 75ml/h. Calculate the amount of D5W she will receive during this period.

To calculate the amount of D5W received by Adeoti you need only to multiply the rate of infusion by the time the pump will be in use.

IV amount = Volumetric pump rate × Time in hours
IV amount = 75ml/h × 10 hours
         = 750ml

Activity 6.4

After a particularly hot day several competitors from various sports have been brought to the surgery where you are working on placement. They are all suffering from dehydration and heat-related stress symptoms. The general practitioner has decided to put them all on *continued . . .* •••

rehydration IV treatment with D5W. Calculate the infusion amount in millilitres that each of the following competitors will receive.

1. Caroline Peates 8 hours at 95ml/h
2. James Pagan 7.5 hours at 105ml/h
3. Jessica Keller 5 hours 45 minutes at 50ml/h
4. Abe Khatun 3 hours 20 minutes at 165ml/h
5. Ciaran O'Rourke 4.25 hours at 75ml/h

At times you may be required to calculate the time a volumetric pump will take to infuse a given amount of fluid at a predetermined or preset rate.

Scenario

Ari Shukla is receiving an infusion of 1.8 litres at the rate of 450ml/h. The consultant treating Ari would like to schedule some further tests for him and has asked you how long this infusion will take.

To calculate the amount of time Ari's IV will take you need to divide the amount to be infused by the rate of the volumetric pump. Since the rate per hour is in millilitres you will first need to convert the amount of the IV to millilitres, then divide this by the rate at which the volumetric pump is to be set.

$$\text{Time in hours for volumetric pump} = \frac{\text{IV in ml}}{\text{Pump rate}}$$

Refer to Chapter 3 (Quantity conversions for nurses) for conversion of litres to millilitres if necessary. Once the amount is converted to millilitres put the figures directly into the formula. The calculation can then be cancelled as shown in Chapter 2, giving the number of hours the volumetric pump will require to infuse the prescribed amount of fluid.

$$\text{Length of time for IV} = \frac{1800}{450}$$

$$= 4 \text{ hours}$$

You can now inform the consultant that the pump will infuse the amount prescribed over four hours.

Activity 6.5

Your placement sees you working in a respite day centre for cancer patients. Some of the patients are due their chemotherapy treatments and these will be given using a number of volumetric pumps. Calculate the time the patients will require to receive their IV amounts.

continued . . .

1. Buster Moves 1 litre at 200ml/h
2. Onya Cycle 2 litres at 500ml/h
3. Rad Casey 1 litre at 400ml/h
4. Rosie Rubberneck 2.5 litres at 750ml/h
5. Thomas La Bengal 2 litres at 250ml/h

There could be times when a patient is ordered an IV amount to be given by volumetric pump in a specific time. In such a scenario you would need to calculate the rate at which the pump should be set to ensure proper timely delivery of the IV amount. This situation might occur if a consultant has prescribed that a new mother is to receive an IV prior to her discharge from the maternity unit or birthing centre.

Scenario

Johanna Stewart is to receive an infusion of 1 litre Lactated Ringer's Solution over a period of 8 hours. You have the volumetric pump prepared and must now determine the rate to deliver the solution over the prescribed time period.

$$\text{IV volumetric pump flow rate} = \frac{\text{IV in ml}}{\text{Hours}}$$

The IV volume is in litres so convert the prescribed volume to millilitres. Refer to Chapter 3 (Quantity conversions for nurses) for conversion of litres to millilitres if necessary. Having converted the amount to millilitres, put the figures into the formula. The calculation will cancel down as shown in Chapter 2 (Essential numeracy requirements for nursing), giving the rate at which the volumetric pump should be set to ensure accurate timely delivery.

$$\text{IV volumetric pump rate} = \frac{1000}{8}$$

$$= 125\text{ml/hour}$$

Activity 6.6

As part of your training you are working in a birthing centre and caring for the new mothers following the birth of their babies. As part of the recovery process the Non Medical Prescribing nurse in charge of the unit has ordered an IV of Lactated Ringer's Solution for the following new mothers. Calculate the rate at which each volumetric pump will be set to ensure the correct flow rate for delivery of the solution in the time prescribed.

1. Busi Adeola 1.25 litres over 4 hours
2. Olivia Campbell 1.35 litres over 4.5 hours

continued . . .

3. Capital Casey 1.1 litres over 2.75 hours
4. Rosy Reynolds 2.5 litres over 6 hours 15 minutes
5. Carolyn Penny 1.8 litres over 6 hours

Chapter summary

An essential skill that every nurse should acquire during their training is accuracy. This chapter has covered the calculation of rates of intravenous infusion to ensure that your patients receive their medication over the prescribed time period. The patient relies on receiving the correct amount of fluid at the correct rate for their recovery and treatment.

The skills you revised in Chapter 3 have been used to convert the required amount of fluid to be given into millilitres; your skills in cancelling down, multiplication, rounding and conversion of time fractions, practised in Chapter 2, have been used to ensure you reach the accurate flow rates.

Answers to the activities

Activity 6.1 (page 91)

1. Thom Flynn 750ml over 8 hours

$$\frac{750 \times 20}{8 \times 60} = 31.2 \text{ giving an IV rate of 31 drops/min}$$

2. Francisca Hall 1.3 litres over 9 hours

$$\frac{1300 \times 20}{9 \times 60} = 48.1 \text{ giving an IV rate of 48 drops/min}$$

3. Simon Cramp 1 litre over 5 hours

$$\frac{1000 \times 20}{5 \times 60} = 66.6 \text{ giving an IV rate of 67 drops/min}$$

4. Kareb Mohamed 500ml over 3 hours

$$\frac{500 \times 20}{3 \times 60} = 55.5 \text{ giving an IV rate of 56 drops/min}$$

5. Poppy Brock 900 millilitres over 5 hours

$$\frac{900 \times 20}{5 \times 60} = 60 \text{ giving an IV rate of 60 drops/min}$$

6. Jessica Wallace $\frac{3}{4}$ litre over $7\frac{1}{2}$ hours

$$\frac{750 \times 20}{7.5 \times 60} = 33.3 \text{ giving an IV rate of 33 drops/min}$$

7. Thomas Major 1.85 litres over a day

$$\frac{1850 \times 20}{24 \times 60} = 25.6 \text{ giving an IV rate of } 26 \text{ drops/min}$$

8. Meow Felinez 750ml over 5 hours 45 minutes

$$\frac{750 \times 20}{5.75 \times 60} = 43.4 \text{ giving an IV rate of } 43 \text{ drops/min}$$

9. Nassir Hussein $1\frac{1}{4}$ litres over 12 hours

$$\frac{1250 \times 20}{12 \times 60} = 34.7 \text{ giving an IV rate of } 35 \text{ drops/min}$$

10. Poppy Seedz 3 litres over 24 hours

$$\frac{3000 \times 20}{24 \times 60} = 41.6 \text{ giving an IV rate of } 42 \text{ drops/min}$$

If necessary, refer to Chapter 3 (Quantity conversions for nurses) for conversion of litres to millilitres, conversion of time, cancelling down and the rounding of fractions and decimals.

Activity 6.2 (page 92)

1. Nigella Faroff 1 litre over 10 hours

$$\frac{1000 \times 15}{10 \times 60} = 25 \text{ giving an IV rate of } 25 \text{ drops/min}$$

2. Wendy Wassit $\frac{1}{2}$ litre over 5 hours

$$\frac{500 \times 15}{10 \times 60} = 25 \text{ giving an IV rate of } 25 \text{ drops/min}$$

3. Alistair Abdul $\frac{3}{4}$ litre over 6 hours

$$\frac{750 \times 15}{6 \times 60} = 31.2 \text{ giving an IV rate of } 31 \text{ drops/min}$$

4. Jodi James 750ml over 5 hours

$$\frac{750 \times 15}{5 \times 60} = 37.5 \text{ giving an IV rate of } 38 \text{ drops/min}$$

5. John Johnstone 250ml over 150 minutes

$$\frac{250 \times 15}{150} = 25 \text{ giving an IV rate of } 25 \text{ drops/min}$$

If necessary, refer to Chapter 3 (Quantity conversions for nurses) for conversion of litres to millilitres, and to Chapter 2 for cancelling down and the rounding of fractions and decimals.

Activity 6.3 (page 93)

$$\text{IV flow rate} = \frac{\text{IV amount in ml} \times \text{giving set}}{\text{Hours} \times 60}$$

1. Ghana Khartoum $\frac{1}{2}$ litre over 5 hours

$$\frac{500 \times 60}{5 \times 60} = 100 \text{ giving an IV rate of } 100 \text{ drops/min}$$

2. Lucy Freeman 200ml over 75 minutes

$$\frac{200 \times 60}{1.25 \times 60} = 160 \text{ giving an IV rate of } 160 \text{ drops/min}$$

3. Linda Peters 0.75 litre over 4 hours

$$\frac{750 \times 60}{4 \times 60} = 187.5 \text{ giving an IV rate of } 188 \text{ drops/min}$$

4. Hilda Hammer 500ml over 6 hours

$$\frac{500 \times 60}{6 \times 60} = 83.3 \text{ giving an IV rate of } 83 \text{ drops/min}$$

5. Carol Johnstone 0.1 litre over 1 hour

$$\frac{100 \times 60}{1 \times 60} = 100 \text{ giving an IV rate of } 100 \text{ drops/min}$$

If necessary, refer to Chapter 3 (Quantity conversions for nurses) for conversion of litres to millilitres if necessary, and to Chapter 2 for cancelling down and the rounding of fractions and decimals.

Activity 6.4 (pages 93–4)

$$\text{IV amount} = \text{Volumetric pump rate} \times \text{Time in hours}$$

1. Caroline Peates 8 hours at 95ml/h so 95×8 gives an infusion of 760ml
2. James Pagan 7.5 hours at 105ml/h so 105×7.5 gives an infusion of 787.5ml
3. Jessica Keller 5 hours 45 minutes at 50ml/h so 50×5.75 gives an infusion of 287.5ml
4. Abe Khatun 3 hours 20 minutes at 165ml/h so $165 \times 3\frac{1}{3}$ gives an infusion of 550ml
5. Ciaran O'Rourke 4.25 hours at 75ml/h so 75×4.25 gives an infusion of 318.75ml

Refer to Chapter 2 for tips on multiplication.

Activity 6.5 (pages 94–5)

$$\text{Time in hours for volumetric pump} = \frac{\text{IV in ml}}{\text{Pump rate}}$$

1. Buster Moves 1 litre at 200ml/h so $1000 \div 200$ will take 5 hours
2. Onya Cycle 2 litres at 500ml/h so $2000 \div 500$ will take 4 hours
3. Rad Casey 1 litre at 400ml/h so $1000 \div 400$ will take 2 hours 30 minutes
4. Rosie Rubberneck 2.5 litre at 750ml/h so $2500 \div 750$ will take 3 hours 20 minutes
5. Thomas La Bengal 2 litres at 250ml/h so $2000 \div 250$ will take 8 hours

If necessary, refer to Chapter 3 (Quantity conversions for nurses) for conversion of litres to millilitres, and to Chapter 2 for cancelling down and the conversion of time fractions or decimals.

Activity 6.6 (pages 95–6)

$$\text{IV volumetric pump flow rate} = \frac{\text{IV in ml}}{\text{Hours}}$$

1. Busi Adeola 1.25 litre over 4 hours so 1250 ÷ 4 will require a rate of 312.5ml/h
2. Olivia Campbell 1.35 litres over 4.5 hours so 1350 ÷ 4.5 will require a rate of 300ml/h
3. Capital Casey 1.1 litres over 2.75 hours so 1100 ÷ 2.5 will require a rate of 400ml/h
4. Rosy Reynolds 2.5 litres over 6 hours 15 minutes so 2500 ÷ 6.25 will require a rate of 400ml/h
5. Carolyn Penny 1.8 litres over 6 hours so 1800 ÷ 6 will require a rate of 300ml/h

Refer to Chapter 2 for cancelling down if necessary.

Useful website

Testandcalc

The following website is useful for IV Flow Rate practice and is free for six months if you register. Try a free download first and register when you need to.

1. IV flow rates quiz
    www.testandcalc.com/quiz/testiv.htm

References

Shivbalan, S, Sathiyasekeran, M and Thomas, K (2010) Therapeutic misadventure with paracetamol in children. *Indian Journal of Pharmacology*, 42: 412–15. Available online at: www.ijp-online.com/text.asp?2010/42/6/412/71894 (accessed 29 May 2012).

Star (2009) *The Star*, 28 November 2009 www.iol.co.za/index.php?set_id=1&click_id=125&art_id=vn20091128082542696C913737 Accessed 30 November 2009

For further activities and other useful material, visit the companion website at **www.sagepub.co.uk/starkings2e**

Chapter 7
Calculations and children

NMC Standards for Pre-registration Nursing Education

At the end of this chapter you will have covered some of the numerical calculations required for the Essential Skills Clusters by the first and second progression point and for entry to the register.

32(2)   Monitors and assesses people receiving intravenous fluids.
33(1)   Is competent in basic medicines calculations.
33(2)   Is competent in the process of medication-related calculation in nursing field
36(4)   Safely manages drug administration and monitors effects.
38(4)   Safely and effectively administers and, where necessary, prepares medicines via routes and methods commonly used and maintains accurate records.

Chapter aims

By the end of this chapter you should be able to:

*   calculate the dose by weight of the child;
*   calculate the dose required by the surface area of a child.

Introduction

You may well recognise that the NMC Standards and **Essential Skills Clusters** for children have already been seen in other chapters of this book. This should come as no surprise as children are in some respects smaller versions of your adult patients. One main difference comes in the range of sizes and weights of child patients, compared to adults. If you are studying Children's Nursing then your patients could range in size from a premature baby as small as 500 grams through to an obese adolescent who may weigh as much as an adult.

The amount of medication an adult patient receives will offer no comparison to that given to a premature baby whose weight has been recorded at 0.52 kilograms. This weight could be as little as $\frac{1}{100}$ of the mother's weight. Complications during the birth could mean that both mother and child require treatment, but the potency of modern drugs and medicines means that the child's dose is not simply $\frac{1}{100}$ of the mother's prescription.

Case study

Maria has given birth to a daughter she has named Friday. The birth was complicated due to Maria having a serious lower respiratory tract infection. During the birth the registrar confirmed that Friday has contracted her mother's infection. Now both Maria and Friday will require treatment for this infection. Maria has an allergy to penicillin and is to be treated with clindamycin. Since Friday is only a few days old and has not yet been tested for any allergic reaction she will be treated with the same drug for now. The drug being used is suitable for both adults and children.

*As an adult, Maria will be treated at a prescribed dose of 450 milligrams given in two equal doses each day for five days. Friday is prescribed a paediatric dosage of 16mg/kg/day in four equal doses, due to her being a small premature baby weighing just 1.35 kilograms. The consultant **paediatrician** could have also prescribed Friday's medication using her body surface area of $0.06m^2$ and a prescription of $360mg/m^2$.*

When prescribing medication for children the dosages are often prescribed according to the patient's weight. This is due to the weight variance of child patients: from a premature baby who may weigh just 500 grams to an obese teenager weighing as much as 60 kilograms or more, child patients can vary greatly in size and weight. Some adult medications are also ordered using the patient's weight; the methods used to calculate these dosages are the same for both adults and children.

By the end of this chapter you should be able to accurately calculate the dosage requirement of any patient, no matter their age, given their weight. As in Chapter 5 (Drug calculations), some activities may require conversion prior to calculation of the dose. These conversions are covered in Chapter 3 (Quantity conversions for nurses) and apply no matter the age or size of your patient. You may wish to revise Chapter 3 as well as Chapter 2 (Essential numeracy requirements for nursing), as both contain essential best-practice skills used in calculating children's medication amounts.

Calculation of dosage by weight

The ability of a nurse to accurately calculate the dosage that a patient under their care is to receive is a fundamental core skill required by all nurses.

Scenario

Bettina McAuliffe is 8 years of age and suffers from focal epileptic seizures. Bettina must take primidone tablets to keep her seizures under control. The tablets have been ordered as 20mg/kg/day to be taken in three equal doses. Bettina weighs 18.75 kilograms. You must calculate the current correct daily dosage amount for this little girl and also how many tablets her mother is to give her for each single dose. Scored tablets of strength 50 milligrams are currently available from the pharmacy supplying Bettina's medication.

In this scenario you will need to use the skills you have practised in the previous chapters. You will use multiplication and division (Chapter 3) and then calculate the number of tablets Bettina's mother will give her daughter each time (Chapter 5).

To calculate Bettina's current daily dosage you must multiply her weight by the amount of milligrams ordered per kilogram.

$$18.75 \times 20 = 375\text{mg}$$

This figure is the daily amount in milligrams that Bettina must take to control her seizures. This total daily dosage will then be divided into the three equal single doses.

$$
\begin{array}{r}
\boxed{1 \quad 2 \quad 5} \\
3 \enclose{longdiv}{3^0 7^1 5}
\end{array}
$$

So Bettina will require 125 milligrams three times daily. You can now calculate the correct number of tablets.

Need = 125mg; Have = 50mg; Stock = 1 tablet

$$\text{The correct dose for Bettina} = \frac{N}{H} \times \frac{S}{1}$$

$$\frac{125}{50} \times \frac{1}{1} = 2\frac{1}{2} \text{ tablets}$$

You can now confidently inform Bettina's mother that the single dose to be taken three times daily will be $2\frac{1}{2}$ tablets.

Hint ... When writing the answer to a drug calculation always remember to include the unit of measure in the answer. This will enable your peers to know exactly the amount of medication and the method of delivery, liquid in millilitres or in tablet form or as capsules, that you have calculated the patient should have, given the individual's prescription.

You should now attempt the following activities without the aid of a calculator.

Activity 7.1

You are on placement with the Community Nurse and attending children who have developed Community-Acquired Pneumonia. The Community Nurse has trained to Non Medical Prescribing status and so is qualified to prescribe medication for the children. All the children range in age from 2 to 10 years and are prescribed 8mg/kg/day of levofloxacin.

Given the weight of each child, how much levofloxacin should each of them be given for their condition?

continued . . .

1. Adam Hooper weighs 14.25kg
2. Ciara Madden weighs 23.65kg
3. Katia Mohamed weighs 15.75kg
4. Michaela Abdulla weighs 23.3kg
5. Andrea Simkins weighs 14.65kg
6. Camille Sympson weighs 17.35kg

Answers to all the activities can be found at the end of the chapter.

Activity 7.2

While you are still on placement with the Community Nurse there is an outbreak of chickenpox. It has been decided that the infected children will be treated with valacyclovir hydrochloride at the dosage of 20mg/kg/day. The medication will be administered by each child's parent or guardian three times daily for five days.

Given the weight of each child, how much valacyclovir hydrochloride should each of them be given as a daily dose for their chickenpox?

1. Simone Mitchell weighs 7.5kg
2. Sean Crampton weighs 24.7kg
3. Mercy Kugani weighs 18.33kg
4. Mohamed Murrumbidg weighs 16.46kg
5. Getaway Zumbia weighs 29.53kg

Activity 7.3

During your studies you have been allocated a placement on the Children's Ward at a major regional hospital. This particular ward specialises in renal patients. As part of their anaemia treatment the children on this ward are being treated with darbepoetin alpha. Each child will receive 2.25mcg/kg by **subcutaneous** injection weekly. Your task at the commencement of today's shift is to calculate the dosage to be drawn up for each child.

1. Harriet Golding weighs 20.6kg
2. Gordon Crucib weighs 5.48kg
3. Tobias Eddy weighs 12.4kg
4. Jax Orbetter weighs 9.56kg
5. Blessing Hearannow weighs 24.16kg

There are some drugs, such as the cancer drug **dactinomycin**, which can be prescribed as either an amount per kilogram of patient weight or as an amount per square metre (m^2) of body surface area (BSA) of the individual patient. In the next activity you are asked to calculate the amount of medication required using a patient's weight. The next section of this chapter covers BSA medication calculations; you will then calculate the drug dosage for the same patients using body surface area rather than weight.

Activity 7.4

The following children are being treated with dactinomycin for a **nephroblastoma**, a tumour of the kidneys that typically occurs in children. The **oncologist** treating the children has prescribed a medication cycle for each child at 15mcg/kg/day. As part of your daily duties you are asked to calculate each child's required dose.

1. Billy Bob Yuall weighs 15.2kg
2. Sam Odeeer weighs 16kg
3. Bethan Charles weighs 28kg
4. Hyacinth Buckerts weighs 26kg
5. Joaquin Johannes weighs 34kg

At the end of the next section these same five children will have their medication prescribed by their body surface area.

Calculation of dosage by surface area

More commonly found in paediatric nursing is dosage by BSA. The BSA of a patient can be found using a commercially available chart known as a **nomogram**. These charts utilise a patient's height and weight to predict or estimate the surface area of the patient's body. Nomograms base the calculation of a patient's BSA on an assumption that the patient is of average weight for their height; obese patients could be measured using other methods. One alternative method of calculating a patient's BSA involves using the Mosteller formula. This formula was first published by the *New England Medical Journal* in 1987 and has been widely reprinted throughout the world in medical journals and texts. It is one of many published formulas that can be used to calculate the BSA of children or adults.

$$\text{BSA (m}^2) = \sqrt{\frac{\text{weight (kg)} \times \text{height (cm)}}{3600}}$$

The Mosteller formula, along with the other even more complex formulas that can be used to calculate a patient's BSA, will not be covered in this book.

The average BSA of children can vary from 0.25m^2 for **neonates** (newborn babies) up to 1.33m^2 for a preteen child. The averages for adults are 1.6m^2 for women and 1.9m^2 for men. With the ongoing development of new drugs to fight diseases, drug delivery methods could change in the future, potentially increasing the practice of prescription by BSA; the skills you practise here could be applied to any patient in your care.

Scenario

Kai Kasugai has acute lymphoblastic leukaemia and is being treated with doxorubicin hydrochloride on a four-weekly cycle of intravenous infusion. Kai has been prescribed a dose of $40mg/m^2$ by his oncologist. With the use of the oncology ward's nomogram you have calculated Kai's body surface area at $1.15m^2$.

You must now calculate the required amount of doxorubicin hydrochloride that he is to receive.

The calculation of dose by BSA is carried out in the same way as the calculation for dose by body weight. So again the skills gained in Chapter 2 (Essential numeracy requirements for nursing) of multiplying decimal numbers will be utilised. Should you feel it necessary, review Chapter 2 before attempting these Chapter 7 activities.

With the use of the nomogram you determined that Kai has a surface area of $1.15m^2$ and the oncologist ordered 40mg for every square metre. Therefore the calculation is 1.15 multiplied by 40.

$$1.15 \times 40 = 46$$

You now know that Kai will require 46mg to be infused during this treatment session. Further treatment, if required, will be determined by his oncologist in 28 days.

Activity 7.5

During this placement you are working at a specialist children's hospital on the cancer ward. The children all attend a special hospital school while staying on the ward and so will be practising their multiplication skills with you. This encourages the children to keep up their studies while in hospital. As with all children, their age, heights and weights are all different and so you must calculate their individual dosages.

The oncologist for the ward is the same as Kai's and has ordered 40mg of doxorubicin hydrochloride for every square metre of BSA for each child. Calculate the correct amount each of the children should receive given their body surface area.

1. Penny Sweetz $0.75m^2$
2. Thomas Llandar $1.48m^2$
3. Iain Trout $0.93m^2$
4. Isabella Mohamed $0.88m^2$
5. Itsa Strange $1.54m^2$

Activity 7.6

Still working with the oncology department, you have moved across to another ward which treats the younger children. These children have been diagnosed with rhabdomyosarcoma, a childhood tumour that usually occurs only in children under five.

continued . . . •

These children are being given vincristine sulfate injections dependent on their body surface area as part of their treatment regime.

The paediatric oncologist has ordered each to be given $1.75mg/m^2$. You are tasked to undertake the calculations to determine each child's dose.

1. Frederica Whittle $0.72m^2$
2. Kareem Hossnian $0.48m^2$
3. Justin Troubell $0.60m^2$
4. Mohamed Mohamed $0.68m^2$
5. Geoff Daimond $0.84m^2$

Activity 7.7

During your extended placement at the specialist children's hospital you have transferred to the paediatric heart ward. In this ward some of the children are suffering from **ventricular arrhythmias** that consultants have diagnosed as life threatening. As these children are all over the age of two they can be treated with sotalol which has been prescribed at $30mg/m^2$ three times daily. You are asked by the Lead Nurse to calculate each child's dose given their individual BSA.

1. Ricardo Turiz $0.57m^2$
2. Eliza Kettle $0.74m^2$
3. Cheryl Persival $0.83m^2$
4. Mader Ingarland $0.92m^2$
5. Woodford Morris $0.675m^2$

The children you met and nursed earlier on the oncology ward are now due their next round of medication. This time the children's doses are to be calculated using their BSA.

Activity 7.8

The following children are being treated with dactinomycin for a nephroblastoma. The oncology registrar treating the children has prescribed an intravenous five-day cycle of treatment for each child at $400mcg/m^2/day$. As part of your daily duties you are asked to calculate each child's required dose. This time their medication will be calculated using each child's BSA.

1. Billy Bob Yuall $0.75m^2$
2. Sam Odeeer $0.6m^2$
3. Bethan Charles $1.05m^2$
4. Hyacinth Buckerts $0.975m^2$
5. Joaquin Johannes $1.275m^2$

Chapter summary

Due to the size and often the fragility of your child patients they are less likely to withstand any inaccuracy in their prescribed medications than adults. Accuracy is an essential, best-practice skill for every nurse, but it is particularly vital in the field of children's or paediatric medication because the values calculated are sometimes very small. Some of the patients you will treat will be too young to tell you where the pain is or that they require something such as a drink or to relieve themselves. These patients will need your best-practice skills and expertise at all times to aid their recovery from ailments or injuries. One day the child you nurse could be your nurse should you require nursing treatment in the future. Set them a good example of how the work of the nurse can improve life for everyone.

Answers to the activities

Activity 7.1 (pages 102–3)

Given the weight of each child and the order for 8mg/kg/day, you need to multiply the weight by 8 to obtain the total daily dosage for each child.

1. Adam Hooper requires $14.25 \times 8 = 114$mg
2. Ciara Madden requires $23.65 \times 8 = 189.2$mg
3. Katia Mohamed requires $15.75 \times 8 = 126$mg
4. Michaela Abdulla requires $23.3 \times 8 = 186.4$mg
5. Andrea Simkins requires $14.65 \times 8 = 117.2$mg
6. Camille Sympson requires $17.35 \times 8 = 138.8$mg

Use the Hint. Whenever writing the answer to a drug calculation always remember to include the unit of measure for the answer. This will enable your peers to know exactly what amount of medication you have calculated that the patient should have.

Activity 7.2 (page 103)

The amount of valacyclovir hydrochloride each child should be given daily for their chickenpox is calculated by multiplying the given weight by the prescribed amount of 20 milligrams per kilogram.

1. Simone Mitchell $7.5 \times 20 = 150$mg
2. Sean Crampton $24.7 \times 20 = 494$mg
3. Mercy Kugani $18.33 \times 20 = 366.6$mg
4. Mohamed Murrumbidg $16.46 \times 20 = 329.2$mg
5. Getaway Zumbia $29.53 \times 20 = 590.6$mg

Remember the Hint and include the unit of measure in your answer to ensure everybody is clear about the exact dose for each patient. Should you feel you need to revise multiplying decimal numbers, refer to Chapter 2 (Essential numeracy requirements for nursing).

Activity 7.3 (page 103)

Each child is to receive 2.25mcg/kg so to calculate the dosage for each child multiply their individual weight by 2.25.

1. Harriet Golding requires 20.6 × 2.25 = 46.35mcg
2. Gordon Crucib requires 5.48 × 2.25 = 12.33mcg
3. Tobias Eddy requires 12.4 × 2.25 = 27.9mcg
4. Jax Orbetter requires 9.56 × 2.25 = 21.51mcg
5. Blessing Hearannow requires 24.16 × 2.25 = 54.36mcg

Remember the Hint and include the unit of measure in your answer to ensure everybody is clear about the exact dose for each patient. Should you feel you need to revise multiplying decimal numbers, refer back to Chapter 2 (Essential numeracy requirements for nursing).

Activity 7.4 (page 104)

For each child to receive 15mcg/kg/day you need to multiply their individual weights by 15.

1. Billy Bob Yuall requires 15.2 × 15 = 228mcg
2. Sam Odeeer requires 16 × 15 = 240mcg
3. Bethan Charles requires 28 × 15 = 420mcg
4. Hyacinth Buckerts requires 26 × 15 = 390mcg
5. Joaquin Johannes requires 34 × 15 = 510mcg

You may wish to revise Chapter 2 (Essential numeracy requirements for nursing) if you have any difficulties with multiplication. Remember the Hint and include the unit of measure in your answers to ensure everybody is clear about the exact dose for each patient.

Activity 7.5 (page 105)

The oncologist has ordered 40mg for every m^2 for each child, so multiply each child's surface area by 40.

1. Penny Sweetz requires 0.75 × 40 = 30mg
2. Thomas Llandar requires 1.48 × 40 = 59.2mg
3. Iain Trout requires 0.93 × 40 = 37.2mg
4. Isabella Mohamed requires 0.88 × 40 = 35.2mg
5. Itsa Strange requires 1.54 × 40 = 61.6mg

Remember the Hint and include the unit of measure in your answer to ensure everybody is clear about the exact dose for each patient. Should you feel you need to revise multiplying decimal numbers, refer to Chapter 2 (Essential numeracy requirements for nursing).

Activity 7.6 (pages 105–6)

The paediatric oncologist ordered 1.75mg/m^2 so multiply each child's surface area by 1.75.

1. Frederica Whittle requires 0.72 × 1.75 = 1.26mg
2. Kareem Hossnian requires 0.48 × 1.75 = 0.84mg
3. Justin Troubell requires 0.60 × 1.75 = 1.05mg
4. Mohamed Mohamed requires 0.68 × 1.75 = 1.19mg
5. Geoff Daimond requires 0.84 × 1.75 = 1.47mg

Revise the multiplication of decimal numbers in Chapter 2 (Essential numeracy requirements for nursing) if you feel it necessary. Remember to include the unit of measure in your answers so your peers are clear about the exact dose for each patient.

Activity 7.7 (page 106)

As the children are being treated with a prescription of $30mg/m^2$, multiply each BSA by 30 to obtain the correct dose.

1. Ricardo Turiz requires $0.57 \times 30 = 17.1mg$
2. Eliza Kettle requires $0.74 \times 30 = 22.2mg$
3. Cheryl Persival requires $0.83 \times 30 = 24.9mg$
4. Mader Ingarland requires $0.92 \times 30 = 27.6mg$
5. Woodford Morris requires $0.675 \times 30 = 20.25mg$

Remember the Hint and include the unit of measure in your answer to ensure everybody is clear about the exact dose for each patient. Should you feel you need to revise multiplying decimal numbers, refer back to Chapter 2 (Essential numeracy requirements for nursing).

Activity 7.8 (page 106)

Each child is to receive $400mcg/m^2/day$, so multiply their BSA by 400 to calculate each child's dose.

1. Billy Bob Yuall requires $0.75 \times 400 = 300mcg$
2. Sam Odeeer requires $0.6 \times 400 = 240mcg$
3. Bethan Charles requires $1.05 \times 400 = 420mcg$
4. Hyacinth Buckerts requires $0.975 \times 400 = 390mcg$
5. Joaquin Johannes requires $1.275 \times 400 = 510mcg$

The daily requirement of each child is the same as that when the dose was calculated using their weight. You may wish to revise the multiplication of decimal numbers using Chapter 2 (Essential numeracy requirements for nursing). Remember to include the unit of measure in your answers to ensure everybody is clear about the exact dose for each patient.

For further activities and other useful material, visit the companion website at **www.sagepub.co.uk/starkings2e**

Chapter 8
Exam skills and revision exercises

Chapter aims

By the end of this chapter you should be able to:

- display the numeracy skills required as a nurse;
- carry out the drug calculations required to administer medicines safely via appropriate routes in Fields of Nursing including specific requirements for children and other groups;
- display the skills required to cancel down fractions as found in nursing calculations;
- multiply decimal numbers by another decimal value as found in nursing calculations;
- divide decimal numbers by another decimal value as found in nursing calculations;

- convert fractions to decimals as found in nursing calculations;
- convert decimals to fractions as found in nursing calculations;
- convert time fractions and decimals to minutes to carry out calculations for nursing;
- round decimal and fraction values as appropriate to nursing calculations;
- convert a given weight, be it of a drug or person, into a greater or lesser unit of weight measure in the metric system of measure as typically found in healthcare;
- convert a liquid measure from litres to millilitres and from millilitres to litres;
- convert a given length into a lesser or greater unit of length measure in the metric system of measurement as typically found in healthcare;
- multiply any amount by 10, 100, 1000;
- record fluid intake as required for healthcare calculations;
- record fluid output as required for healthcare calculations;
- complete a Fluid Balance Chart for patient hydration care;
- provide a fluid balance value for a time period as required to evaluate a patient's hydration level;
- calculate the number of tablets required for patients from their prescription;
- calculate the dose required in liquid form as prescribed for a patient;
- calculate the drug dose prescribed for injection for a patient;
- calculate the drug dose for injection for patients requiring insulin;
- work out the dose to be given to a patient when prescribed by their body weight;
- calculate the flow rate in drops per minute that an intravenous infusion chamber should be set to in order to ensure an accurate delivery flow to individual patients;
- calculate the amount of time required for a volumetric infusion pump to deliver a given volume of fluid to a patient;
- calculate the flow rate required for a volumetric infusion pump to deliver a volume of fluid in a specified amount of time.

Introduction

Revision is an important part of your learning process and hence an essential part of your training. Revision helps to consolidate what you have learnt and should give you a better understanding of the knowledge required of you. Nursing students must pass numeracy and mathematical calculations tests as part of their course to ensure they are competent in these essential skills. There will be other tests of your skills during your training and some subjects are covered in the other books in the Learning Matters series *Transforming Nursing Practice*. This chapter contains some helpful tips and advice to aid your revision gathered from both authors' years of experience as both students and teachers.

Revision techniques

Ideally, the process of revision starts when you first meet the study materials in your class. The easiest way to learn, particularly for nursing calculations, is by doing plenty of examples and asking your tutor(s) questions about any problems as your studies progress. The purpose of revision is to ascertain what you have understood and to consolidate your learning. Here is a list of what you need for revision on any assessed work.

- The up-to-date syllabus for your course that you are being assessed on. This is so you know what is required and can identify all the key areas that will be assessed.
- Your course notes, with any examples given by your tutor. These can be used to help you if you get stuck on a particular topic. Be sure your notes are legible and if necessary rewrite them after the lectures to ensure you understand them. Try using separate folders for each subject to keep them ordered.
- Any text or reference books you have used during the course, especially your copy of *Passing Calculations Tests for Nursing Students*. Having examples of the specialised requirements for your course that can be referred to when needed will be helpful.
- Specimen or past test papers, if available, for the specific course you are following. It is always a good idea to see what has been asked on previous test papers; make sure that any examples you have are related to your course.
- Plenty of pens and paper, and a bottle of water to keep you hydrated.
- Somewhere quiet to do your revision without being interrupted, whether at home, university, a public library or your work place.
- A self-promised reward for yourself at the end of each revision session. It will help to motivate you; all students get fed up at some stage and rewards or an indulgence can often help.

Getting started with revision can be difficult but try to schedule time to revise your coursework regularly. Revision involves you attempting any activity questions or coursework set for your individual course, or just redoing the activities found in this book. Identify the subjects or topics that you feel need revision, then seek help by looking back at your course notes or re-reading the specific chapter in this book. When making your study timetable, remember to put in some revision slots and also some 'you' time when you can enjoy yourself – not too much, though. Half an hour spent revising questions, revisiting chapters in this book or writing down a question you need to ask your tutor is better than two hours spent worrying about what to do, reading aimlessly and hoping some answer will suddenly arrive. You might also find it useful to revise with a friend, to talk problems through and test each other. If so, schedule some time when you can both work together.

The following case studies use the best-practice nursing skills that have been covered in this book. The case studies are based in hospital situations as the majority of nurses do the biggest proportion of their practical training in this environment. Read the following case studies and before attempting to answer the questions ask yourself the following questions.

- Do I understand what is being asked?
- Can I break down each case study into various tasks?

- Can I find all the relevant information here?
- Can I answer all or some of this, or should I revise the relevant chapter(s)?

If you answer yes to all of these, then attempt the case studies in turn. Remember that you can always revise a chapter or chapters in order to grasp the required mathematics. The answers to each case study can be found at the end of the chapter, and will refer you back to relevant chapters should you need further clarification. For example, if you find you are unsure about filling out the Fluid Balance Chart, it is suggested that you revise Chapter 4, then re-attempt the particular case study.

Case study 1: an adult surgical patient with acute anxiety

Mitchell Ahmed has just had major surgery and has arrived on Azalea Ward to regain consciousness from the anaesthetic. As you are on placement in the ward, you will carry out some of his care requirements over the course of your next shifts. Part of your duties today will be to set Mitchell's IV drip rate.

(a) *The surgeon has prescribed 0.5 litre of Hartmann's solution using a 15 drop/ml drip chamber giving set over 5 hours starting at 0800. Calculate the rate that should be set.*

(b) *Create a Fluid Balance Chart for the hours between 8 a.m. and 3 p.m. given the following fluid measurements taken. Mitchell is also receiving an IV of one litre Lactated Ringer's solution being given over a period of 16 hours. The IV is currently being infused using a 15 drop/ml drip chamber giving set and was commenced at 8 a.m. Be sure to include the intravenous drip (IV) he is receiving in your calculations.*

0800	Tea	65ml		
0915			Urine	165ml
1000			Vomit	235ml
1030	Juice	55ml		
1230			Urine	200ml
1300	Water	75ml		
1400			Urine	215ml
1415			Vomit	105ml
1430	Tea	50ml		

What is Mitchell's fluid balance in litres?

(c) *What time is Mitchell's IV of Lactated Ringer's solution due to be completed?*

(d) *What is the correct rate for this drip chamber giving set to ensure this is achieved?*

(e) *Mitchell is experiencing severe discomfort following his surgery, and the registrar has prescribed apomorphine. The prescription states he should receive 4 milligrams of apomorphine. The drug is available on Azalea Ward in strength of 0.02g/ml. You must now calculate the correct dose to be given to Mitchell.*

(f) *Mitchell is to receive donepezil for his anxiety ongoing condition at the rate of 3mg/day given b.i.d. The medication is available in either 0.5mg or 1mg tablets. Calculate what combination of tablets Mitchell requires. Donepezil tablets should not be broken and should be given only as whole tablets.*

continued . . .

(g)   It is found that Mitchell has an E coli infection and it is to be treated with kanamycin. The kanamycin is to be given intramuscularly and is prescribed on body weight. Mitchell was weighed on admission and this was recorded as 75 kilograms. The consultant has prescribed 15mg/kg/day given in two equal doses. The drug is available in strength 1g/4ml and you are asked to calculate the amount of each single dose.

The next case study takes elements of the mathematical calculations from throughout this book which are required as best practice by all nurses.

Case study 2: a small child patient

Carolyn Cent (date of birth 1 February 2007 and NHS Number BY 14623P) is a six-year-old girl diagnosed with leukaemia, and she has been admitted to Woodlands Hospital Peony Ward for her next chemotherapy treatment. She has a body surface area of 0.8m² and her weight of 20 kilograms was recorded on admission.

As part of your nursing training you are on placement in the ward where Carolyn is currently being treated. As part of your placement you will later join the community nurse who will visit Carolyn at home for follow-up care.

Carolyn is to be treated using two different drugs for this round of medication. You are to be part of her primary care team and at the start of this shift must calculate the amount of each drug she is to receive.

(a)   *The first drug Carolyn will receive is teniposide prescribed at the amount of 165mg/m². The teniposide is available on your ward in stock strength 50mg/5ml. How much of the drug is Carolyn to receive?*

(b)   *The second drug prescribed in the treatment of Carolyn's acute lymphoblastic leukaemia is cytarabine at the amount of 300mg/m². The drug has been reconstituted and is available in stock strength 100mg/ml. How much cytarabine should Carolyn receive by subcutaneous injection?*

(c)   *Given the following recordings of fluid intake, prepare a Fluid Balance Chart for Carolyn for the hours 7 a.m. until 12 noon.*

Carolyn is reluctant to take fluids orally so her paediatric oncologist has ordered an intravenous drip (IV) to ensure she maintains a healthy fluid balance. Carolyn will receive 625ml of Dextrose 5% using a drip chamber giving set of 20 drops/ml over 5 hours. The IV will start at 9 a.m. and run continuously for the 5 hours prescribed by the oncologist.

Time	Intake	Amount	Output	Amount
0715	Water	110ml		
0730			Urine	250ml
0830	Juice	200ml		
0900			Urine	175ml
0915			Vomit	300ml
0930	Juice	150ml		
1000			Vomit	90ml
1030	Water	120ml		
1200			Urine	200ml

continued . . . •••

What is Carolyn's fluid balance in millilitres for this time period?

(d)   *What rate should the drip chamber giving set be to ensure correct delivery of Carolyn's IV?*

Following her treatment at the hospital Carolyn is now home and receiving ongoing treatments. Your placement at the hospital has also now been completed and you have moved to the community clinic. This clinic is the one that Carolyn's home-visiting non-medical prescribing (NMP) nurse works from, so you will accompany her on visits to Carolyn at home.

(e)   *As well as leukaemia Carolyn also suffers grand mal seizures, and this condition is kept under control through the use of medication.*

Carolyn takes primidone for her seizures and has been prescribed 15mg/kg/day. The primidone is in tablet form and available in stock strength 50 milligrams. If Carolyn is to take her seizure medication three times a day, how many tablets should she take per dose?

(f)   *Because of the side effects of the primidone Carolyn's mother gives her supplementary doses of folic acid. The tablets are stock strength 0.4 milligrams. What is 0.4 milligrams as micrograms?*

(g)   *On a later visit to Carolyn's home you find that, having returned to school, she has contracted chickenpox from an unknown source. The NMP is currently dealing with many of these cases in her community and so prescribes acyclovir to treat Carolyn. The prescription is for 80mg/kg/day given four times daily. As Carolyn already takes many tablets, the NMP suggests a liquid form of the drug. This banana-flavoured medication is available in stock strength 0.2g/5ml. How much acyclovir should Carolyn take per single dose?*

(h)   *As Carolyn has fully recovered from her bout of chickenpox her mother has agreed to allow Carolyn on a trip to her grandmother's home in the Lake District for five days. Her mother has asked you how much acyclovir Carolyn will need to take with her for the 5-day trip. What amount will you tell her?*

Exam tips

The exam tips listed below give some advice on how to survive and do well in assessments tasks.

✓ Always check your learning timetable for any assessments. You need to know what time it is to be taken or submitted.
✓ If you are going to do a written assessment, always organise yourself regarding what you need to submit or take with you. For example, have your identity card, pens and pencils ready to hand.
✓ Arrive at least 10 minutes early at the assessment centre for any written test.
✓ Before undertaking any of your assessed tasks, have a good night's sleep, making sure you have a reliable alarm clock or someone to wake you up in plenty of time.
✓ Have something to eat and allow lots of time to travel, leaving early to be sure of arriving on time.
✓ Remember to listen to and/or read any instructions given to you by the invigilators and answer every question as fully as you can.

✓ Attempt all the questions required, taking careful note of the time you have allowed for each question. Do not spend too long on any one question.

✓ Move to another question if you get stuck on a particular question as you can always come back to this question if you have time before the end of the examination.

✓ Some examinations will give you a choice of what questions to answer, so make sure you read the instructions on the number of questions – you may not have to do them all.

✓ See assessments as a chance to show off what you know; by now you have done plenty of revision and practice questions.

✓ Promise yourself a reward after the assessment so you have something to look forward to afterwards. I always found this was a good motivator for me!

Chapter summary

This chapter covers a variety of numerical and mathematical tasks which nurses and other nurses may be required to perform. By the time you reach this part of the book you should have done some revision and are ready to do your coursework-assessed tasks.

Good luck with your assessments and, on behalf of all your prospective patients and service users, we thank you for caring for us.

Answers to the case studies

Case study 1 (page 113)

(a) Mitchell is to receive an IV of 0.5 litre of Hartmann's solution using a 15 drop/ml drip chamber giving set over 5 hours. You are to determine the drip rate at which the giving set should be set.

The calculation of IV rates is covered in Chapter 6 (Calculating intravenous rates), and you should refer back to this for revision.

$$\text{IV flow rate} = \frac{\text{IV amount in ml} \times \text{giving set}}{\text{Hours} \times 60}$$

$$\text{IV rate} = \frac{500 \times 15}{5 \times 60} = 25$$

This figure does not need to be rounded. As seen in Chapter 2, if the decimal is over halfway, the amount will be rounded up.

Answer: IV rate 25 drops/minute

(b) You are asked to create a Fluid Balance Chart for the hours between 8 a.m. and 3 p.m. Be sure to include the intravenous drip (IV) he is receiving in your calculations.

An example of a Fluid Balance Chart is shown in Chapter 4.

Remember that Mitchell is also receiving a litre of IV fluid over 16 hours. This requires you to calculate how much fluid is infused each hour, so you should refer to Chapter 2 (Essential numeracy requirements for nursing) for revision. Since 1 litre equals 1000 millilitres you will need to divide 1000ml by 16 to obtain the number of millilitres per hour. Refer to Chapter 2 for the division of numbers revision, and to Chapter 3 (Quantity conversions for nurses) for revision on conversion of litres to millilitres.

$$\text{IV amount per hour} = \frac{1000}{16} = 62.5\text{ml}$$

Answer: IV rate 62.5ml/hour

This figure must appear each hour on your Fluid Balance Chart as it is part of Mitchell's fluid intake.

Woodland Hospital	Clinical Skills Fluid Balance Chart
Ward: Azalea	Date: 21/03/2013 M/F: M
Family Name: Ahmed	First Name: Mitchell
NHS Number: AC 14351L	Date of Birth: 01/04/1957

	INTAKE				OUTPUT				
Time	By Mouth or Tube	ml	Intravenous	ml	Urine ml	Vomit or Tube	ml	Other	ml
0700									
0800	Tea	65	IV Fluid	162.5					
0900			IV Fluid	162.5	165				
1000	Juice	55	IV Fluid	162.5		Vomit	235		
1100			IV Fluid	162.5					
1200			IV Fluid	162.5	200				
1300	Water	75	IV Fluid	62.5					
1400	Tea	50	IV Fluid	62.5	215	Vomit	105		
1500			IV Fluid	62.5					
1600									
Totals		245		1000	580		340		
Total Input 0800–1500: 1245ml					**Total Output 0700–1500:** 920ml				
Fluid Balance for time period = +325ml									

You are asked to calculate Mitchell's fluid balance in millilitres. Fluid balance was covered in Chapter 4 (Fluid balance and maintenance), and you should refer back to it for revision if needed.

Fluid balance = Total input − Total output

Total input = 65 + 162.5 + 162.5 + 162.5 + 55 + 162.5 + 162.5 + 75 + 62.5 + 50 + 62.5 + 62.5 = 1245

Total output = 165 + 235 + 200 + 215 + 105 = 920

Therefore Mitchell has a fluid balance of 1245 − 920 = +325ml

Answer: Positive 0.325 litre fluid balance

(c) Mitchell's IV of Lactated Ringer's solution is due to be completed 16 hours after it was started. Since it was started at 8 a.m. – which is 0800 – you need to add 16 hours to this figure. This means the IV is scheduled to complete at midnight, which is 0000hrs.

Answer: midnight or 0000hrs

(d) You are asked to calculate the correct rate for the drip chamber giving set to ensure that the IV schedule is completed in the correct time schedule.

The calculation of IV rates is covered in Chapter 6 (Calculating intravenous rates), and you should refer back to this for revision.

$$\text{IV flow rate} = \frac{\text{IV amount in ml} \times \text{giving set}}{\text{Hours} \times 60}$$

$$\text{IV rate} = \frac{1000 \times 15}{16 \times 60} = 15.6 \text{ drops/minute}$$

The cancelling down of fractions was covered in Chapter 2 (Essential numeracy requirements for nursing). The result above must now be rounded (also covered in Chapter 2). As the decimal is over halfway, the amount will be rounded up. You may wish to revise Chapter 2 for both these skills.

Answer: IV rate 16 drops/minute

(e) Mitchell is prescribed 4 milligrams of apomorphine from a stock strength of 0.02g/ml. You are asked to calculate the correct dose to be given to Mitchell.

The calculation of drug dosages was covered in Chapter 5, and if needed, you should refer to it for revision practice. You may also want to revise Chapter 3 (Quantity conversions for nurses), as one of the given amounts in this question will need converting.

0.02g/ml = 20mg/ml

Now to the actual dosage calculation.

Need 4mg   **H**ave 20mg   **S**tock 1ml

$$\frac{N}{H} \times \frac{S}{1} = \text{The correct dose for the patient}$$

$$\frac{4}{20} \times \frac{1}{1} = 0.2\text{ml}$$

(Remember to put the unit of measure in your answer.)

The cancelling down of fractions was covered in Chapter 2 (Essential numeracy requirements for nursing), and you may wish to revise this chapter.

Answer: 0.2ml of apomorphine is the correct dose for Mitchell

(f) Mitchell is to receive donepezil that has been prescribed at 3mg/ day given b.i.d. You are asked to calculate the combination of tablets he is to receive given the drug is available in strength 0.5mg and 1 mg tablets.

Mitchell requires 3 milligrams of donepezil b.i.d – which means two equal doses given daily. Therefore each dose should be 3 ÷ 2 = 1.5mg per dose.

The calculation of drug dosages was covered in Chapter 5, and if needed, you should refer to it for revision practice. Since the tablets come in strengths of 0.5mg and 1mg, the most obvious combination for Mitchell would be one of each tablet. This combination would allow for the least number of tablets for Mitchell each time. Remember the advice that donepezil tablets are not to be broken before administration to patients; some tablets could allow for the patient to be given half-tablets, so be sure to check all medication and never assume the conditions of administration for any medication.

Answer: 1 × 1mg tablet + 1 × 0.5mg tablet gives the correct dose with the least number of tablets

(g) The consultant has prescribed kanamycin at 15mg/kg/day to be given in two equal doses. The drug is available in strength 1g/4ml and you are tasked to calculate the amount of each single dose. Mitchell was weighed on admission, and this was recorded as 75 kilograms.

Dosage of a patient using their weight was covered in Chapter 7 (Calculations and children). Given Mitchell has a recorded weight of 75 kilograms and was prescribed 15 milligrams for each kilogram, the calculation to find his required dose is:

$75 \times 15 = 1125$mg

The multiplication of numbers was covered in Chapter 2 (Essential numeracy requirements for nursing).

You now know Mitchell requires 1125 milligrams of kanamycin and must calculate the amount to be given.

You may also want to revise Chapter 3 (Quantity conversions for nurses), as one of the given amounts will need converting in this question.

1g/4ml = 1000mg/4ml

Now calculate of the required dosage amount.

Need 1125mg   **H**ave 1000mg   **S**tock 4ml

$$\frac{N}{H} \times \frac{S}{1} = \text{The correct dose for the patient}$$

$$\frac{1125}{1000} \times \frac{4}{1} = 4.5\text{ml}$$

(Remember to put the unit of measure in your answer.)

The cancelling down of fractions was covered in Chapter 2 (Essential numeracy requirements for nursing), and you may wish to revise this chapter.

You have calculated that Mitchell will take 4.5 millilitres per day, but this will be given over 2 equal doses. In order to calculate a single dose, divide the daily requirement by the number of equal doses to be given.

$4.5 \div 2 = 2.25$

You now have the amount required for each single dose for Mitchell.

Answer: 2.25ml per dose

Case study 2 (pages 114–15)

(a) Carolyn will receive teniposide prescribed at the amount of 165mg/m². In Chapter 7 (Calculations and children), you revised how to calculate the dose a patient requires given their BSA. Carolyn has a BSA of 0.8m². To calculate her dosage, you need to multiply her BSA by the prescribed dose.

$0.8 \times 165 = 132$mg

Now that you have the required amount, you can calculate the required dose given the stock strength available on the ward. You practised this calculation in Chapter 5 (Drug calculations).

Since the teniposide is available on your ward in stock strength 50mg/5ml the calculation, will look like this.

Need 132mg   **H**ave 50mg   **S**tock 5ml

$$\frac{N}{H} \times \frac{S}{1} = \text{The correct dose for the patient}$$

$$\frac{132}{50} \times \frac{5}{1} = 13.2\text{ml}$$

(Remember to put the unit of measure in your answer.)

The cancelling down of fractions was covered in Chapter 2 (Essential numeracy requirements for nursing), and you may wish to revise this chapter.

Answer: 13.2ml

(b) The other treatment Carolyn has been prescribed is cytarabine given at the amount of 300mg/m^2. Again, in Chapter 7 (Calculations and children), you revised how to calculate the dose a patient requires given their BSA. Carolyn has a BSA of 0.8m^2. To calculate her dosage, you need to multiply her BSA by the prescribed dose.

$$0.8 \text{ x } 300 = 240\text{mg}$$

Now that you have the required amount, you can calculate the required dose given the stock strength available on the ward. You practised this calculation in Chapter 5 (Drug calculations).

Since the cytarabine has been reconstituted and is available in stock strength 100mg/ml the calculation will look like this:

Need 240mg   **H**ave 100mg   **S**tock 1ml

$$\frac{N}{H} \times \frac{S}{1} = \text{The correct dose for the patient}$$

$$\frac{240}{100} \times \frac{1}{1} = 2.4\text{ml}$$

(Remember to put the unit of measure in your answer.)

The cancelling down of fractions was covered in Chapter 2 (Essential numeracy requirements for nursing), and you may wish to revise this chapter.

Answer: 2.4ml

(c) The Fluid Balance Chart for Carolyn between the hours of 7 a.m. and 12 noon given fluid measurements taken should look like the chart below. Be sure to include in your chart the intravenous drip (IV) she is receiving.

Carolyn is to receive 625 millilitres of IV fluid over 5 hours starting at 9 a.m. So you will need to calculate how much fluid is infused during each hour for the period being recorded. Refer to Chapter 2 (Essential numeracy requirements for nursing) for the division of numbers revision.

$$\text{IV amount per hour} = \frac{625}{5} = 125\text{ml}$$

This amount of fluid must appear each hour on your fluid balance chart as it is part of Carolyn's fluid intake.

Look at the fluid balance chart to calculate Carolyn's fluid balance in millilitres between the hours required. Total all of her inputs and outputs, including the IV amounts relevant to the time frame. Fluid balance was covered in Chapter 4 (Fluid balance and maintenance), and you should refer back to it for revision if needed.

Fluid balance = Total input − Total output

Total input = 110 + 200 + 125 + 150 + 125 + 120 + 125 + 125 = 1080

	Woodland Hospital		Clinical Skills Fluid Balance Chart
	Ward: Peony		Date: 21/03/2013 M/F: F
	Family Name: Cent		First Name: Carolyn
	NHS Number: BY 14623P		Date of Birth: 01/02/2007

| Time | INTAKE | | | | OUTPUT | | | | |
	By Mouth or Tube	ml	Intravenous	ml	Urine ml	Vomit or Tube	ml	Other	ml
0600									
0700	Water	110			250				
0800	Juice	200							
0900	Tea	150	Dextrose 5%	125	175	Vomit	300		
1000	Water	120	Dextrose 5%	125		Vomit	90		
1100			Dextrose 5%	125					
1200			Dextrose 5%	125	200				
1300			Dextrose 5%	125					
1400									
Totals	580			625	625	390			
Total Input 0700–1200: 1080ml					**Total Output 0700–1200:** 1015ml				
Fluid Balance for time period = +65ml									

Total output = 250 + 175 + 300 + 90 + 200 = 1015

Therefore Carolyn has a fluid balance of 1080 − 1015 = 65ml

Answer: +65ml fluid balance

(d) You are asked to calculate the correct rate for the drip chamber giving set to ensure Carolyn receives her IV in the prescribed time period.

The calculation of IV rates is covered in Chapter 6 (Calculating intravenous rates), and you should refer back to this for revision.

$$\text{IV flow rate} = \frac{\text{IV amount in ml} \times \text{giving set}}{\text{Hours} \times 60}$$

$$\text{IV rate} = \frac{625 \times 20}{5 \times 60} = 41\frac{2}{3} \rightarrow 42 \text{ drops/minute}$$

The cancelling down of fractions was covered in Chapter 2 (Essential numeracy requirements for nursing).

Answer: IV rate 42 drops/minute

(e) Carolyn's seizure medication is prescribed in an amount per kilogram of weight. Her weight of 20 kilograms was recorded on admission. Her consultant has prescribed primidone at 15mg/kg/day to be given in three equal doses. The drug is available in strength 50 milligram tablets and you are tasked to calculate the amount of each single dose. First, calculate the amount in milligrams she will require given her weight.

$20 \times 15 = 300$ milligrams

The multiplication of numbers was covered in Chapter 2 (Essential numeracy requirements for nursing).

You now know that Carolyn requires 300 milligrams of primidone and must calculate the required dosage amount.

Need 300mg   **H**ave 50mg   **S**tock 1 tablet

$$\frac{N}{H} \times \frac{S}{1} = \text{The correct dose for the patient}$$

$$\frac{300}{50} \times \frac{1}{1} = 6 \text{ tablets/day}$$

(Remember to put the unit of measure in your answer.)

The cancelling down of fractions was covered in Chapter 2 (Essential numeracy requirements for nursing), and you may wish to revise this chapter.

You have calculated that Carolyn will take 6 tablets per day, but this will be given over 3 equal doses. In order to calculate a single dose, divide the daily requirement by the number of equal doses to be given.

$6 \div 3 = 2$

You now have the amount required for each single dose for Carolyn.

Answer: 2 tablets per dose

(f) Because of the side effects of one of medications, Carolyn takes a folic acid supplement. The tablets are of strength 0.4 milligrams and you are asked for this amount in micrograms. In Chapter 3 (Quantity conversions for nurses), you learnt how to do the conversion. You may wish to review this chapter for revision. Using the ladder found in Chapter 3 you know that micrograms are below milligrams and to move down is to multiply. Multiply is to move the decimal point right three places and so your conversion should look like this:

0 4 0 0.

Carolyn's folic acid supplements are 400 micrograms in strength.

Answer: 400 micrograms

(g) Some people you meet seem to have terrible luck when it comes to health, and Carolyn is one of those people, but she does not complain. Now she has chickenpox and needs acyclovir to treat it. The community nurse you are working with on placement has prescribed 80mg/kg/day in four equal doses.

First calculate the amount in milligrams she will require given her weight.

$20 \times 80 = 1600$ milligrams

The multiplication of numbers was covered in Chapter 2 (Essential numeracy requirements for nursing).

You now know Carolyn requires 1600 milligrams of acyclovir and must calculate the amount to be given.

You may also want to revise Chapter 3 (Quantity conversions for nurses), as one of the given amounts will need converting in this question.

0.2g/5ml = 200mg/5ml

Now calculate of the required dosage amount.

Need 1600mg   **H**ave 200mg   **S**tock 5ml

$$\frac{N}{H} \times \frac{S}{1} = \text{The correct dose for the patient}$$

$$\frac{1600}{200} \times \frac{5}{1} = 40 \text{ millilitres/day}$$

(Remember to put the unit of measure in your answer.)

The cancelling down of fractions was covered in Chapter 2 (Essential numeracy requirements for nursing), and you may wish to revise this chapter.

You have calculated that Carolyn will take 40 millilitres per day, but this will be given over 4 equal doses. In order to calculate a single dose, divide the daily requirement by the number of equal doses to be given.

$40 \div 4 = 10$ millilitres

You now have the amount required for each single dose for Carolyn.

Answer: 10 millilitres per dose

(h) Carolyn is looking forward to her trip to her grandmother's house, and you are calculating the amount of acyclovir she must take with her. Given that she takes 10 millilitres per dose 4 times daily you can calculate her daily amount. However, you have already done this in part (g) and know it to be 40 millilitres. All that remains for you to do is to multiply the daily requirement by the five days of her holiday. The multiplication of numbers was covered in Chapter 2 (Essential numeracy requirements for nursing).

$40 \times 5 = 200$ millilitres

Answer: 200 millilitres required for the 5-day trip

Remember to wish Carolyn good luck on her trip just as the authors wish you good luck with your training, studies and your career as a registered nurse.

Useful websites

BBC Bitesize and Mathcentre

The BBC Bitesize and the HEA Mathcentre online resources offer revision material that you can use to enhance your numeracy skills. The web pages for each of the chapters you need to revise can be found at the end of those chapters.

Testandcalc

This website is useful for drug calculations practice and is free for six months if you register. Try a free download first and register when you need to.

1.   Metric conversions quiz
     www.testandcalc.com/quiz/testmet.htm

2. Fluid dosages quiz
   www.testandcalc.com/quiz/testflu.htm

3. IV flow rates quiz
   www.testandcalc.com/quiz/testiv.htm

4. Tablet dosages quiz
   www.testandcalc.com/quiz/testtab.htm

Nursing Standard

The *Nursing Standard* nursing journal offers online guides and resources for you free of charge. The following two, among others, relate to drug calculations.

5. Improving the numeracy skills of nurse prescribers
   http://nursingstandard.rcnpublishing.co.uk/resources/archive/GetArticleById.asp?ArticleId=4534

6. Drug calculations part 1: a critique of the formula used by nurses
   http://nursingstandard.rcnpublishing.co.uk/resources/archive/GetArticleById.asp?ArticleId=6542

MSOR

The Maths, Stats and OR Network has produced the following Study Skills for the Mathematical Sciences.

7. Study skills leaflet
   www.mathstore.ac.uk/repository/studyskillsleaflet.pdf

For further activities and other useful material, visit the companion website at
www.sagepub.co.uk/starkings2e

Glossary

Dactinomycin: A highly toxic drug used in chemotherapy regimens for the treatment of renal cancer in children.

Drip chamber: The use of a drip chamber allows an estimate of the rate at which fluid is administered for an IV infusion.

Essential Skills Clusters: Skills and behaviours that students will need to demonstrate in order to prove achievement in specified competencies.

Fluid balance: The difference between fluid input and fluid output.

Fluid Balance Chart(s): Records a patient's hourly fluid intake and output over a specified time period.

Fluid intake: The amount of fluid a patient consumes via oral drinks, food, intravenous fluids or tube feeds.

Fluid output: The amount of fluid a patient excretes via urine, vomiting, tube drainage, diarrhoea, gastric secretions or wound drainage.

Giving set: A device used to break down the flow of each millilitre of fluid, from an IV infusion, into droplets.

Injection/Intravenous infusion: An injection is an infusion method of putting fluid into the body, usually with a hollow needle and a syringe which is pierced through the skin to force fluid into a vein or tissue.

Macrodrip: A chamber that coverts each millilitre of fluid, from an IV infusion, into 15 or 20 drops.

Microdrip: A chamber that converts each millilitre of fluid, from an IV infusion, into 60 drops.

Neonate: A small child or baby.

Nephroblastoma: Tumour of the kidneys found mostly in children; also known as Wilms' Tumour.

Nomogram: A graphical calculating device, a two-dimensional diagram designed to allow the approximate graphical computation of a function, in this case the surface area of a human body.

Oncologist: A medical professional who practises oncology; oncology is a branch of medicine that deals with tumours (cancer).

Orally: By mouth (e.g. many drugs are taken orally).

Paediatrician: A doctor or consultant who deals with the medical care of infants, children and adolescents.

Paediatrics: The branch of medicine that deals with the medical care of infants, children and adolescents.

Plasma: Blood plasma is the yellow liquid component of blood, in which the blood cells in whole blood would normally be suspended.

Platelets: These are small, irregularly shaped anuclear cells (i.e. cells that do not have a nucleus containing DNA) which form clots in blood.

Prime number: A number which is exactly divisible by only 1 and itself.

Registrar: A medical doctor in the UK receiving advanced training in a specialist field.

Stock strength or dispensed dose: The amount of drug as kept in a specified strength in the pharmacy or on the ward in the medicine cabinet.

Strength required or prescribed strength: The amount of drug to be given to the patient.

Subcutaneous: An injection administered as a bolus into the subcutis, which is the layer of skin directly below the dermis and epidermis.

Ventricular arrhythmias: A condition in which there is abnormal activity in the heart.

Volumetric pump: A pump that is used to deliver rates of fluid intravenously at 5ml or more per hour.

Drug calculations

N is for **Need**; **H** is for **Have**; **S** is for the **stock volume**

Put them together and you get

$$\frac{N}{H} \times \frac{S}{1} = \text{The correct dose for the patient}$$

The ladder to Successful Nursing

IV rate calculation

$$\frac{\text{Amount of IV in millilitres} \times \text{giving set}}{\text{Number of hours} \times 60} = \text{Number of drops per minute}$$

The ladder for height conversion

Index